Handbook of
Targeted Cancer Therapy
and Immunotherapy

Gastrointestinal Cancer

Handbook of
Targeted Cancer Therapy and Immunotherapy
Gastrointestinal Cancer

Editors

Milind Javle, MD
Professor
Division of Cancer Medicine
Department of Gastrointestinal Medical Oncology
The University of Texas MD Anderson Cancer Center
Houston, Texas

Mitesh J. Borad, MD
Professor of Medicine
Mayo Clinic College of Medicine and Science
Mayo Clinic Comprehensive Cancer Center
Phoenix, Arizona

Series Editors

Daniel D. Karp, MD
Professor of Medicine
Department of Investigational Cancer Therapeutics
Principal Investigator of the MD Anderson Clinical & Translational Science Award (CTSA)
The University of Texas MD Anderson Cancer Center
Houston, Texas

Gerald S. Falchook, MD, MS
Director
Drug Development Unit
Sarah Cannon Research Institute at HealthONE
Presbyterian/St. Luke's Medical Center
Denver, Colorado

JoAnn D. Lim, PharmD, BCOP
Clinical Pharmacy Specialist, Phase I
Division of Pharmacy
Department of Investigational Cancer Therapeutics
The University of Texas MD Anderson Cancer Center
Houston, Texas

🔵 Wolters Kluwer

Philadelphia • Baltimore • New York • London
Buenos Aires • Hong Kong • Sydney • Tokyo

Acquisitions Editor: Joe Cho
Development Editor: Eric McDermott
Editorial Coordinator: Priyanka Alagar
Marketing Manager: Phyllis Hitner
Production Project Manager: Catherine Ott
Manager, Graphic Arts & Design: Stephen Druding
Manufacturing Coordinator: Lisa Bowling
Prepress Vendor: S4Carlisle Publishing Services

9 8 7 6 5 4 3 2 1

Printed in Mexico

Library of Congress Cataloging-in-Publication Data

ISBN-13: 978-1-975162-94-8

Cataloging in Publication data available on request from publisher.

shop.lww.com

QUADM0723

Contributors

Kavitha Balaji, PhD
AstraZeneca

Sarah Baldwin, RN, ANP-BC, BSN, MSN
The University of Texas MD Anderson Cancer Center

Tamara G. Barnes, RN, MSN, CNS, AOCNS
The University of Texas MD Anderson Cancer Center

Laura Beatty, PA-C
The University of Texas MD Anderson Cancer Center

Tanios Bekaii-Saab, MD
Mayo Clinic

Lindsay Gaido Bramwell, MSN, RN, ACNS-BC
Flatiron Health

Sara Bresser, MPAS, PA-C
The University of Texas MD Anderson Cancer Center

Amanda Brink, DNP, APRN, FNP-BC, AOCNP
The University of Texas MD Anderson Cancer Center

Isabel Cepeda, MSN, RN, AGN-P
The University of Texas MD Anderson Cancer Center

Ian Chau, MD
Royal Marsden Hospital

Arvind Dasari, MD, MS
The University of Texas MD Anderson Cancer Center

Timothy Philip DiPeri, MD
The University of Texas MD Anderson Cancer Center

Ecaterina Dumbrava, MD
The University of Texas MD Anderson Cancer Center

Ben George, MD
Medical College of Wisconsin

Roman Groisberg, MD
Rutgers Cancer Institute of New Jersey

Thorvardur R. Halfdanarson, MD
Mayo Clinic

Daniel M. Halperin, MD
The University of Texas MD Anderson Cancer Center

Nicholas James Hornstein, MD
The University of Texas MD Anderson Cancer Center

Ryan Huey, MD
The University of Texas MD Anderson Cancer Center

Filip Janku, MD, PhD
The University of Texas MD Anderson Cancer Center

Milind Javle, MD
The University of Texas MD Anderson Cancer Center

Daniel D. Karp, MD
The University of Texas MD Anderson Cancer Center

Ahmed O. Kaseb, MD
The University of Texas MD Anderson Cancer Center

Ed Kheder, MD
The University of Texas MD Anderson Cancer Center

Holly Kinahan, RN, MSN, NP-C, AOCNP
The University of Texas MD Anderson Cancer Center

Michael Sangmin Lee, MD
The University of Texas MD Anderson Cancer Center

Sunyoung S. Lee, MD
The University of Texas MD Anderson Cancer Center

Gregory B. Lesinski, PhD, MPH
Emory University

JoAnn D. Lim, PharmD, BCOP
The University of Texas MD Anderson Cancer Center

Shalini Makawita, MD
Baylor College of Medicine

Kathrina Marcelo-Lewis, PhD
The University of Texas MD Anderson Cancer Center

Hossein Maymani, MD
Rocky Mountain Cancer Centers

Funda Meric-Bernstam, MD
The University of Texas MD Anderson
Cancer Center

Sandra Montez, RN
The University of Texas MD Anderson Cancer Center

Shyamm Moorthy, PhD
The University of Texas MD Anderson Cancer Center

Van Karlyle Morris, MD
The University of Texas MD Anderson Cancer Center

Justin Moyers, MD
The University of Texas MD Anderson Cancer Center
University of California, Irvine College of Medicine

Shubham Pant, MD
The University of Texas MD Anderson Cancer Center

Christine Parseghian, MD
The University of Texas MD Anderson Cancer Center

Amy B. Patel, MPAS, PA-C
The University of Texas MD Anderson Cancer Center

Maggie Phillips, BSc
Emory University

Rille Pihlak, MD, PhD
The Royal Marsden NHS Foundation Trust

Patrick Pilie, MD
The University of Texas MD Anderson Cancer Center

viii

Kanwal Pratap Sing Raghav, MD
The University of Texas MD Anderson
Cancer Center

Matthew J. Reilley, MD
University of Virginia

Jordi Rodon-Ahnert, MD, PhD
The University of Texas MD Anderson Cancer Center

Shiraj Sen, MD, PhD

Ana Stuckett, PhD
The University of Texas MD Anderson Cancer Center

Gabriele Urschel, DNP, RN, FNP-C, AOCNP
The University of Texas MD Anderson Cancer Center

Irene S. Yu, MD
The University of Texas MD Anderson Cancer Center

Preface

Precision medicine, also referred to as "personalized medicine," has led to transformative changes for patients with gastrointestinal malignancies over the past decade. The advent of next-generation sequencing, liquid biopsies, identification of cellular signaling pathways across different cancer types, and nimble mechanisms for drug development has contributed to this success. It is essential that scientific advances and novel therapeutics be easily accessible to the practicing clinician who is making quick decisions based on the clinical and molecular data. We are building on the success of *Handbook of Targeted Cancer Therapy and Immunotherapy* and are pleased to present a focused *Handbook of Targeted Cancer Therapy and Immunotherapy: Gastrointestinal Cancer* in a similar format. Our hope is that this book will provide a quick and easy reference guide for management decisions in the clinic. Each chapter includes a short summary of targeted therapy approaches followed by a table of molecular targets and potential therapies as applicable to the individual cancer type along with relevant citations. We recognize that several of the proposed therapies lack level one evidence from phase III clinical trials, may need further validation, and should therefore be considered judiciously. Providing both a succinct and comprehensive review on different cancer types is certainly challenging, particularly when the field is changing rapidly. We were fortunate to have some of the leaders in the field coauthor this book and are extremely grateful for their contributions. Patients and their families are our inspiration and we look forward to making cancer history with them!

Milind Javle, MD
Mitesh J. Borad, MD

Acknowledgments

We are indebted to Wolters Kluwer Health for guiding us through this process and for their patience. We also thank Drs Dan Karp and Gerald Falchook for this opportunity.

x

Contents

SECTION 1 Targets by Organ Site 1
Milind Javle and Mitesh Borad, Editors

CHAPTER 1 Colorectal Cancer 2
Christine Parseghian

CHAPTER 2 **Gastric and Esophageal Cancer** 18

Rille Pihlak and Ian Chau

CHAPTER 3 **Liver Cancer (Hepatocellular)** 28

Irene S. Yu and Ahmed O. Kaseb

SECTION 2 **Sequencing Technologies** 85
Milind Javle, Editor

CHAPTER 9 **Introduction of High-Throughput Sequencing** 86
Timothy Philip DiPeri and Funda Meric-Bernstam

CHAPTER 10 **Liquid Biopsies in Gastrointestinal Cancers** 93
Shalini Makawita and Arvind Dasari

SECTION 4 **Targeted and Immunotherapy Agents** 223

JoAnn D. Lim and Justin Moyers, Editors
Sarah Baldwin, Tamara G. Barnes, Laura Beatty, Sara Bresser,
Amanda Brink, Isabel Cepeda, Lindsay Gaido Bramwell,
Holly Kinahan, JoAnn D. Lim, Justin Moyers, Amy B. Patel, and
Gabriele Urschel, Contributors

Targets by Organ Site

CHAPTER 1

Colorectal Cancer

Christine Parseghian

Targeting RAS

CETUXIMAB

Cetuximab is a chimeric immunoglobulin G1 (IgG1) monoclonal antibody directed against the epidermal growth factor receptor (*EGFR*). It does not benefit patients with metastatic colorectal cancer (mCRC) with oncogenic *RAS* mutations (1). The *KRAS* mutation was initially identified in codons 12 and 13 of exon 2, which result in constitutive activation of the RAS-RAF-MEK-ERK (MAPK) pathway (2–4). Activating mutations in *KRAS* are detected in approximately 40% of mCRC with good concordance between primary tumors and distant metastases of mCRC (5–7). Expanded *RAS* mutations in *KRAS* exon 3 or 4, or in *NRAS* exon 2, 3, or 4 have also been noted to predict a lack of benefit from anti-EGFR therapy (EGFRi), increasing the prevalence of all innate *RAS* mutations to 50% to 55% (2,8,9).

In a phase III trial of cetuximab monotherapy vs. best supportive care (BSC), patients with refractory KRAS wild type (WT) mCRC receiving cetuximab had a relative risk (RR) of 13% compared to 1% in patients with mutant KRAS (codons 12/13). Patients with KRAS WT CRC receiving cetuximab monotherapy vs. those receiving BSC experienced a longer progression-free survival (PFS) (3.7 vs. 1.9 months) and longer overall survival (OS) (9.5 vs. 4.8 months) (1). In the phase III FIRE-3 trial, KRAS/NRAS WT patients receiving FOLFIRI + cetuximab in the frontline setting experienced a RR of 72%, a PFS of 10.3 months, and an OS of 33.1 months, compared to 56%, 10.2 months, and 25 months, respectively, in KRAS/NRAS WT patients receiving FOLFIRI + bevacizumab.

The most significant toxicities associated with cetuximab include diarrhea, hypomagnesemia, hypocalcemia, and an acneiform rash. Traditionally, the risk of an allergic hypersensitivity reaction is reported to be <5%. However, life-threatening anaphylactic hypersensitivity reactions have been reported in up to 30% of patients residing in select geographic locations (10).

Cetuximab is currently U.S. Food and Drug Administration (FDA) approved as monotherapy for patients with mCRC who are intolerant of irinotecan-based regimens or in combination with irinotecan after progression of disease. The findings of the CRYSTAL trial also led to the approval of cetuximab in the frontline setting.

PANITUMUMAB

Panitumumab is a fully human IgG2 monoclonal antibody directed against *EGFR*. In a randomized phase III trial, patients with refractory metastatic disease received BSC with or without panitumumab. In KRAS WT patients, RR was 16% compared to 1% in patients with KRAS MT (mutated). In patients with KRAS, NRAS, and BRAF WT, RR was 18%. In patients with KRAS WT, but mutations in either NRAS or BRAF, the RR was 0% (11). Thus, panitumumab is now FDA approved as a single agent for patients failing irinotecan- and oxaliplatin-based chemotherapy. In another phase III trial, patients treated in the frontline setting with FOLFOX/FOLFIRI with or without panitumumab achieved an improvement in PFS and OS compared to the control arm (PFS 10 vs. 8.6 months, and OS 23.9 vs. 19.7 months) (12). This trial led to the FDA approval of panitumumab in combination with FOLFOX or FOLFIRI in the first- or second-line setting. A large randomized phase II trial (ASPECCT) (*N* = 1010) found that panitumumab is noninferior to cetuximab (*Z* score −3.19; *p* = 0.0007) and that these agents provide similar OS benefit in patients with chemotherapy-refractory disease (10.0 vs. 10.4 months, respectively) (13). Infusion reactions are uncommon with panitumumab because it is a fully humanized monoclonal antibody.

Targeting VEGF/VEGFR

REGORAFENIB

Regorafenib, a small-molecule inhibitor of multiple kinases that is involved with various processes including tumor growth and angiogenesis, has documented efficacy in a salvage therapy setting in mCRC. The phase III CORRECT trial randomized 760 patients who progressed on standard therapy to BSC or regorafenib. The trial met its primary endpoint of OS (6.4 vs. 5.0 months for regorafenib and placebo, respectively; hazard ratio [HR], 0.77; *p* = 0.005). PFS was also significantly but modestly improved (1.9 vs. 1.7 months; *p* < 0.000001) (14). Regorafenib is FDA approved as a salvage therapy option in patients with mCRC who have previously been treated with 5-fluorouracil (5-FU), oxaliplatin, irinotecan, a vascular endothelial growth factor (VEGF) inhibitor, and, if RAS WT, anti-EGFR therapy. It can be given before or after trifluridine-tipiracil in the third-line setting, as no data inform the best order of these therapies.

Unfortunately, although response rates to regorafenib are low, adverse events are high. The most common severe toxicities observed with regorafenib were hand–foot skin reaction, fatigue, diarrhea, and hypertension. In a meta-analysis of four studies, the incidence of all-grade hand–foot skin reactions in 500 patients with CRC was 46.6% (15). To address this, the phase II ReDOS trial investigated the use of an alternative dosing schedule to reduce the toxicities related to regorafenib treatment. Rates of several of the most common adverse events were lower among the dose-escalation group compared to the standard dosing group. Based on these results, the dose-escalation strategy is an appropriate alternative approach for regorafenib dosing (16).

BEVACIZUMAB

Bevacizumab is a humanized monoclonal antibody that binds all isoforms of circulating VEGF, thereby inhibiting permeability and angiogenesis mediated by this factor. In a phase III trial in previously untreated mCRC, patients were randomly assigned either to receive irinotecan, bolus fluorouracil, and leucovorin (IFL) + bevacizumab or IFL + placebo. The median duration of survival was 20.3 months in the group given IFL + bevacizumab, as compared with 15.6 months in the group given IFL + placebo, corresponding to a HR for death of 0.66 ($p < 0.001$). The median PFS was 10.6 months in the group given IFL + bevacizumab, as compared with 6.2 months in the group given IFL + placebo. The corresponding rates of response were 45% and 35%, respectively ($p = 0.004$). The median duration of response (mDOR) was 10.4 months in the group given IFL + bevacizumab, as compared with 7.1 months in the group given IFL + placebo ($p = 0.001$). Grade 3 hypertension was more common during treatment with IFL + bevacizumab than with IFL + placebo (11.0% vs. 2.3%) but was easily managed (17). Bevacizumab is thus FDA approved for use in combination with fluorouracil-based regimens as a first- or second-line treatment for mCRC. Because bevacizumab has essentially no clinical activity as monotherapy in CRC, it cannot be recommended as a single agent and should not be considered for adjuvant therapy outside a clinical trial.

Targeting BRAF V600E Mutations

BRAF is a serine threonine kinase that is downstream of RAS in the MAPK pathway and is mutually exclusive from concurrent *RAS* mutations (18). The most common BRAF mutation occurs at codon 600 with a valine to glutamic acid change (c.1799T>A or p.V600E), producing a constitutively active protein (19,20). In clinical practice, approximately 5% to 8% of all mCRC carries a BRAF V600E mutation and this portends a poor prognosis (21–24). Patients with BRAF V600E mCRC have a distinct clinical presentation accompanied with hallmark pathologic features that include older females, right-sided T4 tumors, high-grade mucinous histology, sporadic microsatellite instability-high (MSI-H) phenotype, and predominantly distal nodal involvement with peritoneal disease (25–27).

In the setting of their aggressive nature and comparatively short survival in patients with BRAF V600E mutations, the initial therapeutic decisions are paramount for patients presenting with metastatic disease. There are data to support the utilization of triplet chemotherapy in combination with bevacizumab for BRAF V600E mCRC based on the TRIBE study that compared FOLFOXIRI + bevacizumab vs. FOLFIRI + bevacizumab for treatment-naïve mCRC (28). In this study, the primary endpoint of PFS was met with an improvement of 2.4 months for all patients that received the triplet regimen compared to doublet. In regard specifically to BRAF V600E, 28 patients were included in this trial, of whom 16 were randomized to the triplet arm. Subgroup analysis revealed that the triplet regimen resulted in improvement of OS to 19 months, compared to 10.7 months with the doublet regimen (28). Therefore, in the first-line setting for BRAF V600E mCRC patients with adequate performance status, FOLFOXIRI in addition to bevacizumab is a reasonable treatment choice. Of note, in this same study the RAS/RAF WT cohort that received triplet therapy had a median OS of nearly 42 months, highlighting the innate aggressiveness of BRAF V600E MT mCRC.

Distinct from melanoma, reactivation of EGFR signaling is the most prominent mechanism of resistance in mCRC after single-agent BRAF inhibition, supporting the development of rational combination therapies (29,30). Initial clinical studies exploring the efficacy of BRAF and EGFR targeted therapies revealed disease response in 52% and 67% of treatment-refractory patients, respectively (31,32). Most notably, when this dual targeted approach was combined with chemotherapy (vemurafenib, irinotecan, cetuximab) in the SWOG 1406 study, superior PFS (4.4 vs. 2.0 months) and overall response rate (ORR) (16% vs. 4%) were achieved among patients exposed to the three-drug combination arm compared to those who received irinotecan and cetuximab alone (33), supporting its initial insertion into treatment guidelines.

The first randomized phase III trial for previously treated BRAF V600E mCRC, known as the BEACON trial, has been completed and published with updated survival data reported (34). This pivotal trial evaluated the efficacy of a BRAF inhibitor encorafenib + cetuximab, with or without the MEK inhibitor binimetinib in comparison to the control arm of irinotecan/FOLFIRI +

cetuximab. Initial safety lead in data reported an ORR of 48% with good tolerability among 29 patients who received the triplet regimen (35). Interestingly, updated survival data revealed that the doublet regimen (encorafenib + cetuximab) was no less efficacious than the triplet regimen. The doublet arm revealed an improved median OS of 8.4 months compared with 5.4 months for the control arm (HR 0.60, $p = 0.0003$) as well as an improved median PFS of 4.2 months compared with 1.5 months for control (HR 0.40, $p < 0.0001$). Additionally, ORR was noted to be 20% for the doublet arm compared to 2% with control ($p < 0.0001$) (34). Based on these data, FDA approval was granted for the doublet regimen in the refractory setting.

Targeting HER2 Overexpression

Human epidermal growth factor receptor (HER2) is a member of the EGFR receptor family and aberrant signaling is known to occur via genomic amplifications promoting upregulation of phosphoinositide 3-kinase (PI3K) and MAPK pathways (36). In CRC, *HER2* amplification is noted in 3% to 5% of patients and may be associated with de novo resistance to EGFR monoclonal antibodies (37). In breast cancer, HER2 amplifications occur at an increased frequency and have been the focus of therapeutic targeting via monoclonal antibodies, trastuzumab and pertuzumab. Serving as a precedent, this approach was pursued in CRC trials with success. The HERACLES trial accrued CRC patients with HER2 positivity defined as 3+ HER2 score in >50% of tumor cells by immunohistochemistry or with 2+ HER2 score and a HER2:CEP17 ratio >2 in >50% of cells by fluorescence in situ hybridization (FISH). In this study, trastuzumab in combination with lapatinib (an oral dual HER2/EGFR kinase inhibitor) was used to treat 27 patients with refractory HER2 mCRC. Nearly 30% of patients had an objective response, with one patient developing a complete response (38). In the phase II MyPathway study, 57 refractory HER2-amplified mCRC patients were treated with a combination dual-HER2 targeted approach of pertuzumab and trastuzumab, revealing a 32% ORR and one patient with a complete response (39). Considering these two positive landmark studies, the NCCN has added HER2 targeted therapy with trastuzumab and lapatinib or trastuzumab and pertuzumab as viable options for patients with refractory HER2-amplified mCRC. Based on early reports of HER2 amplification representing a negative predictive biomarker for EGFR monoclonal antibodies, we await results from the ongoing phase II SWOG 1613 study (NCT03365882) evaluating patients with chemotherapy-refractory, anti-EGFR-naïve HER2-amplified, RAS/RAF WT mCRC randomizing to trastuzumab/pertuzumab vs. cetuximab and irinotecan.

Targeting NTRK Fusions

Neurotrophic tyrosine receptor kinase (NTRK) fusion genes encode for TrkA, TrkB, and TrkC receptor tyrosine kinases that are responsible for baseline function in human neuronal tissue with activation via MAPK and PI3K pathways (40). Fusions can be aberrant, resulting in oncogenic addiction with a rare prevalence of 0.2% to 2.4% of all CRC, with data suggesting higher rates, approaching 3%, in the MSI-H subpopulation (41). It is important to highlight the landmark trial evaluating the efficacy of larotrectinib, a highly selective small-molecule inhibitor of TRK proteins for patients with NTRK fusions (42). In this study, 55 adult and pediatric patients achieved an ORR of 75%, with 55% of patients remaining progression free at 1 year. Among three patients enrolled with CRC, two achieved an objective response. In several phase I/II trials studying an alternative NTRK inhibitor, entrectinib, the ORR across all tumor types was 57% in the refractory setting, with a 7% CR rate. Among CRC patients, RR was 25%. These data have resulted in FDA accelerated tissue-agnostic approval to utilize larotrectinib or entrectinib for all patients with refractory solid tumors and an NTRK fusion. The NCCN has since recommended testing for NTRK gene fusions in mCRC and support the administration of larotrectinib or entrectinib for this rare cohort of patients. Of note, the approval of larotrectinib and entrectinib for patients with NTRK fusions irrespective of cancer histology represents only the second tissue-agnostic FDA drug approval in the era of precision medicine.

Targeting MSI-H mCRC

Deficient mismatch repair (dMMR) or MSI-H accounts for only 4% to 5% of all patients with mCRC; however, it represents a unique cohort with a distinct prognosis and treatment option in the form of immunotherapy (43,44). During the process of DNA replication, repetitive DNA sequences found in our genome known as microsatellites are prone to errors in insertion and deletions. Mismatched errors that occur between the primer and template strands in a microsatellite are normally resolved via the mismatch repair (MMR) system; however, if defective, replicative mistakes ensue, resulting in hypermutations and MSI (45). Considering the hypermutated phenotype of dMMR tumors, the utilization of checkpoint inhibitors has offered an exciting new treatment strategy for patients with mCRC. Targeting programmed death ligand 1 (PD-L1) on tumor cells or programmed cell death 1 (PD-1) protein on T cells has dramatically impacted patient outcomes. Pembrolizumab and nivolumab are two IgG4 monoclonal antibodies that target PD-1, and are both FDA approved for MSI-H mCRC after demonstrating durable clinical activity. The CHECKMATE-142 study investigated the use of nivolumab alone or in combination with ipilimumab, a fully human IgG1 monoclonal antibody that targets cytotoxic T-cell lymphocyte antigen-4 (CTLA-4). In the monotherapy arm, the ORR was 31.3%, with nearly 70% of patients achieving disease control at 12 weeks and a median OS of 73% at 1 year (46). In the doublet arm, whereas grade 3 to 4 treatment-related adverse events increased (32%), the ORR was 55% with a disease control rate (DCR) of 80% and a 1-year OS of 85% (47). Single-agent data for pembrolizumab was first reported in a landmark phase II study investigating its efficacy among 41 patients with refractory, advanced CRC with or without mismatch-repair deficiency (44). Both immune-related ORR and PFS were noted to be 40% and 78%, respectively, among patients with dMMR mCRC compared to 0% and 11% for pMMR mCRC. At the time of the report, the median PFS and OS were not reached for the dMMR cohort and 2.2 and 5.0 months for the pMMR cohort, respectively. More recently, pembrolizumab was also evaluated in the frontline setting in patients with dMMR mCRC. In the KEYNOTE-177 study, pembrolizumab was compared to the investigator's choice of FOLFOX or FOLFIRI and/or bevacizumab or cetuximab in the frontline setting. ORR for pembrolizumab was 45.1% compared to 33.1% in the chemotherapy arm. Median PFS was 16.5 vs. 8.2 months and OS benefit was not found; however, there was a high crossover rate (60%) limiting this analysis (48). Based on these findings, pembrolizumab is now approved by the FDA for dMMR CRC in the frontline setting.

Based on the data, MSI status is a definitive predictive biomarker for response to immune checkpoint blockade. Both NCCN and ESMO guidelines mandate universal testing for MMR or MSI status in order to facilitate diagnosis of patients with Lynch syndrome, provide guidance for patients with stage II CRC, and identify those patients for whom immunotherapy will be efficacious in the metastatic setting. NCCN has included single-agent pembrolizumab, nivolumab, or nivolumab + ipilimumab as viable treatment options for patients with dMMR mCRC in a second- or third-line setting as well as those deemed "not appropriate for intensive therapy" (21,22).

Targeting Ultramutators: POLE and High Tumor Mutational Burden

The POLE gene is located in 12q24.33 and encodes the proofreading exonuclease domain of polymerase epsilon (49). Somatic mutations in *POLE* are a rare event in CRC, estimated at <1%, while mutually exclusive from dMMR (50). Deciphering between passenger and driver *POLE* mutations is of importance in regard to predicting successful outcomes with checkpoint inhibition (51). However, *POLE* mutations are important to highlight considering patients with these mutations have an increased rate of hypermutated tumors (tumor mutational burden [TMB] ≥10 mutations/megabase [TMB-H]) with higher neoantigen load, thereby potentially representing a predictive biomarker for immunotherapy in pMMR CRC (52). In a retrospective cohort, RR to PD1/PD-L1 inhibition in patients with somatic POLE MTs was 27% (53). In a separate retrospective analysis of patients from KEYNOTE-158 who had various previously treated unresectable or metastatic TMB-H solid tumors and were receiving pembrolizumab, there was an ORR of 34.3% and a 9.9% CR rate. The median DOR was not reached, with 58% of patients having response durations ≥12 months and 14% of patients having response durations ≥24 months (54). Thus, although immunotherapy in patients with POLE mutations is not yet FDA approved, based on results of the KEYNOTE-158 trial, patients with TMB ≥ 10 mutations/megabase now have an FDA-approved indication for the use of pembrolizumab in the refractory setting.

Actionable Target	Abnormality	Prevalence (%)	Clinical Experience with Targeted Agent
BRAF	Mutation	5–8	**Vemurafenib** (BRAF inhibitor): • Phase 2, with cetuximab (EGFR inhibitor) and irinotecan: PFS 4.3 vs. 2.0 months (HR 0.48), PR 17% vs. 4%, DCR (PR + SD) 65% vs. 21% favoring the arm with vemurafenib (55) **Dabrafenib** (BRAF inhibitor): • Phase 1/2, with trametinib and panitumumab: RR and SD of 10% and 90% for dabrafenib + panitumumab, 0% and 55% for trametinib + panitumumab, and 21% and 68% for dabrafenib + trametinib + panitumumab (56) **Encorafenib** (BRAF inhibitor) (FDA approved): • Phase 3, with cetuximab (EGFR inhibitor) ± binimetinib (MEK inhibitor) vs. chemotherapy: RR 26% vs. 2%, OS 9.0 vs. 5.4 months (HR 0.52; $P < 0.001$) in BRAF V600E mutated CRC pts who had progressed on 1 or 2 prior regimens (57)

(continued)

Actionable Target	Abnormality	Prevalence (%)	Clinical Experience with Targeted Agent
			• Phase 2, with cetuximab (EGFR inhibitor) + binimetinib (MEK inhibitor) vs. chemotherapy: RR 50%, PFS 4.9 months in first line (58)
HER2 (ERBB2)	Amplification	2–11	**Trastuzumab** (HER2 inhibitor) + **lapatinib** (HER2 inhibitor/EGFR inhibitor): • Phase 2: RR 30%, PR 26%, including 1 (4%) CR, SD 44%, in pts with refractory KRAS WT and HER2-amplified/overexpressed (38) **Pertuzumab** (HER2 inhibitor) + **Trastuzumab** (HER2 inhibitor): • Phase 2a: RR 32%, PR 30%, including 1 (2%) CR in pts with refractory KRAS WT and HER2-amplified/overexpressed (39) **Traztuzumab-deruxtecan** (HER2 inhibitor): • Phase 2: RR 45.3%, including 1 CR and 23 PRs; median duration of response was not reached (59).

Actionable Target	Abnormality	Prevalence (%)	Clinical Experience with Targeted Agent
KRAS G12C		1–3	**Sotorasib** (KRAS^{G12C} Inhibitor): • Phase 1: RR 7.1%, DCR 73.8%, and PFS 4.0 months in the subgroup of mCRC harboring the *KRAS* p.G12C mutation in third-line or later setting (60). • Phase 1b/2, + panitumumab (EGFR inhibitor): RR 27%, DCR 81% in previously treated mCRC (61). **Adagrasib** (KRAS^{G12C} Inhibitor): • Phase 1/2, monotherapy: RR 22%, DCR 87% in 2nd line and later (62). • Phase 1/2 + cetuximab (EGFR inhibitor): RR 43%, DCR 100% in 2nd line and later (62).
MSI-H, dMMR	Loss of at least one mismatch repair protein by IHC (MSH2, MLH1, MSH6, PMS2), or MSI-H by PCR or NGS assay	15 (5 of stage IV)	**Pembrolizumab** (PD-1 inhibitor) (FDA approved for pts with MSI-H or dMMR including mCRC in first line): • Phase 3, monotherapy in first line: 16.5 vs. 8.2 months, RR 43.8% vs. 33.1% compared with chemotherapy (48)

(*continued*)

Actionable Target	Abnormality	Prevalence (%)	Clinical Experience with Targeted Agent
			Nivolumab (PD-1 inhibitor) (FDA approved for pts with MSI-H or dMMR including mCRC in second line): • Phase 2, monotherapy: RR 31%, DCR 69% in MSI-H tumors in pretreated patients with dMMR/MSI-H (46) • Phase 2, + ipilimumab (CTLA4 inhibitor) PR and SD of 52.4% and 31% in MSI-H tumors • Phase 2 + ipilimumab (CTLA4 inhibitor) in first line: RR 69%, PFS and OS not reached (63) **Atezolizumab** (PD-L1 inhibitor): • Phase 1b, with bevacizumab: RR 30% and SD 60% in MSI-H pts (64)
POLE	Abnormality	1	**PD-1/PD-L1 inhibitors:** in a retrospective cohort, **RR** 27% to PD-1/PD-L1 inhibition (53)

Actionable Target	Abnormality	Prevalence (%)	Clinical Experience with Targeted Agent
NTRK	Fusion		**Entrectinib** (FDA approved 2019) (TRK inhibitor): • Phase 1/2 (STARTRK-2, STARTRK-1, ALKA-372-001): ORR 57% across all tumor types (95% CI 43–71), including a 7% complete response rate. RR 25% in colorectal cancer pts (65) **Larotrectinib** (FDA approved 2018) (TRK inhibitor): • Phase 1/2: ORR 79% across all tumor types, CR 24 pts, PR 97 pts, SD 19 pts. RR 50% in colorectal cancer pts (42)
RAS (KRAS/ NRAS)	Mutation (resistance)	30–50	**Cetuximab** (EGFR inhibitor) (FDA approved): • Phase 3, monotherapy: RR 13% in WT KRAS vs. 1% in mutant KRAS (codons 12/13). PFS (3.7 vs. 1.9 months) and OS (9.5 vs. 4.8 months) favored cetuximab compared with BSC in WT KRAS. No difference in mutant KRAS pts (1). • Phase 3: RR 72%, PFS 10.3 months, OS 33.1 months in first-line setting associated with chemotherapy in WT KRAS and NRAS (10)

(*continued*)

Actionable Target	Abnormality	Prevalence (%)	Clinical Experience with Targeted Agent
			Panitumumab (EGFR inhibitor) (FDA approved): • Phase 3, monotherapy: RR 16% in WT KRAS vs. 1% in mutant KRAS. In pts with WT KRAS, NRAS, and BRAF, RR 18%. In pts with WT KRAS and mutations in NRAS or BRAF, RR 0% (11) • Phase 3: PFS 10.0 vs. 8.6 months, OS 23.9 vs. 19.7 months with chemotherapy in KRAS WT pts on first-line setting (12)
VEGF/VEGFR			**Regorafenib** (VEGFR inhibitor) (FDA approved): • Phase 3, monotherapy: OS 6.4 vs. 5.0 months, PFS 1.9 vs. 1.7 months. RR 1% vs. 0.4% compared with placebo (14) **Ramucirumab** (VEGFR2 inhibitor): • Phase 3: OS 13.3 vs. 11.7 months, PFS 5.7 vs. 4.5 months, RR 13.4% vs. 12.5% in association with chemotherapy compared with placebo + chemotherapy (66)

Actionable Target	Abnormality	Prevalence (%)	Clinical Experience with Targeted Agent
			Bevacizumab (VEGF inhibitor) (FDA approved): • Phase 3: RR 45% vs. 35%, OS 20 vs. 16 months; TTP 11 vs. 6.0 months with chemotherapy in first line (17) **Aflibercept** (VEGF inhibitor) (FDA approved): • Phase 3: RR 19.8% vs. 11.1% placebo, OS 13.5 vs. 12.1 months placebo; PFS 6.9 vs. 4.7 months placebo with chemo in second line (67) **Anlotinib** (VEGFR inhibitor) (FDA approved): • Phase 3, monotherapy: OS 8.6 vs. 7.2, PFS 4.1 vs. 1.5 months, RR 4.3% vs. 0.7%, DCR 75.9% vs. 30.7%, compared to placebo in refractory mCRC (68).

BRAF, B-Raf proto-oncogene; BSC, best supportive care; CI, confidence interval; CR, Complete response; CRC, colorectal cancer; DCR, disease control rate; DOR, duration of response; dMMR, deficient mismatch repair; EGFR, epidermal growth factor receptor; FDA, Food and Drug Administration; HER2, human epidermal growth factor receptor 2; HR, hazard ratio; IHS, immunohistochemistry; KRAS, KRAS proto-oncogene; MEK, mitogen activated protein kinase-kinase; MSI-H, microsatellite instability high; NGS, next-generation sequencing; NRAS, neuroblastoma ras viral oncogene homolog; ORR, objective response rate; OS, overall survival; PCR, polymerase chain reaction; PD-1, programmed cell death 1; PD-L1, programmed death-ligand 1; PFS, progression-free survival; PR, partial response; RAS, rat sarcoma virus; RR, response rate; SD, stable disease; TRK, tropomyosin receptor kinase; TTP, time to progression; VEGFR, vascular endothelial growth factor receptor; WT, wild type

CHAPTER 2

Gastric and Esophageal Cancer

Rille Pihlak and Ian Chau

Introduction

Gastric (G), gastroesophageal junction (GOJ), and esophageal (O) cancers are common cancers responsible for >1 million cases diagnosed globally in 2020 (1), making gastric cancer fifth and esophageal cancer seventh most common cancers (1). These are also aggressive cancers with median overall survival (OS) ranging around 1 year in the advanced setting. Standard of care treatment for advanced upper gastrointestinal cancers has been platinum- and fluoropyrimidine-based combination chemotherapy with or without human epidermal growth factor receptor 2 (HER2)-targeted agents for a long time. Recently, various clinical trials have shown the potential benefit of adding immunotherapy to standard of care chemotherapy to improve outcomes.

Currently targeted therapy for G/GOJ/O cancers is mainly based on HER2, microsatellite instability (MSI), and more recently programmed death-ligand 1 (PD-L1) status. However, smaller numbers of other molecular targets are being investigated in various clinical trials with some early promising results.

HER2

Over a decade ago, the phase III ToGA trial showed benefit of targeting HER2 in patients with HER2$^+$ advanced G/GOJ cancers in the first-line setting (2):

- HER2$^+$ present in around 15% to 25% of patients with advanced G/GOJ cancers
- Trastuzumab (HER2 inhibitor) vs. placebo combined with cisplatin and 5-fluorouracil (FU)/capecitabine—median OS improvement by 2.7 months (13.8 vs. 11.1 months)
- HER2 testing by immunohistochemistry (IHC) became a biomarker for advanced G/GOJ cancers directing treatment in the first-line setting.

Recent phase II DESTINY-Gastric01 trial showed efficacy of trastuzumab deruxtecan (HER2 antibody–drug conjugate with a topoisomerase I inhibitor) in the third-line setting or beyond (3):

- Previously trastuzumab treated, progressing after at least two lines of treatment
- Compared to physician choice of standard chemotherapy

- Trastuzumab deruxtecan vs. chemotherapy—ORR 51% vs. 14%; OS 12.5 vs. 8.4 months, respectively (3)
- Preferably repeat HER2 testing on tissue required after first-line trastuzumab treatment to confirm HER2 positivity.

PD-L1

Various immunotherapy trials in G/GOJ/O cancers have investigated PD-L1 status as a potential predictive biomarker:

- Methods assessing PD-L1 expression and the cut-off levels vary between trials.
- Combined positive score (CPS) is the most commonly used method, with cut-offs of CPS ≥ 5 and CPS ≥ 10 being used.

Esophageal cancer:

- In first-line advanced esophageal cancer, the phase III Keynote 590 trial with cisplatin, 5-FU, and pembrolizumab (PD-1 antibody) or placebo showed an improvement in median OS for all patients by 2.5 months (12.4 vs. 9.8 months) and the effect was strongest in the squamous cell carcinoma (SCC) subgroup with CPS ≥ 10 (13.9 vs. 8.8 months) (4).
- The CheckMate 648 trial included only esophageal SCC and showed benefit of adding nivolumab (anti-PD-1) to standard chemotherapy with 5-FU and cisplatin compared to nivolumab + ipilimumab (anti-CTLA-4) or chemotherapy alone. The predictive biomarker used in this study was the tumor cell PD-L1 $\geq 1\%$, which was present in around 48% of patients and in that subgroup, the addition of nivolumab to standard of care chemotherapy showed a median OS improvement by 6.3 months (15.4 vs. 9.1 months) (5).

Gastric cancer:

- The phase III CheckMate 649 trial included first-line patients with advanced gastric, GOJ, and esophageal adenocarcinomas and investigated the addition of nivolumab to standard doublet chemotherapy compared to placebo. The predictive biomarker used in the trial was CPS ≥ 5 and this was present in around 62% of patients in the study. In that subgroup of patients, the median

OS difference was 3.3 months (14.4 vs. 11.1 months), whereas in all patients this was 2.2 months (13.8 vs. 11.6 months) (6).

- Another phase III ORIENT-16 trial also confirmed the addition of sintilimab (PD-1 inhibitor) to oxaliplatin and capecitabine significantly improved OS (7). Similarly, CPS ≥5 was present in 61% of patients (7).

FGFR

Fibroblast growth factor receptor 2 (FGFR2) overexpression and gene amplifications have been found in gastric/GOJ cancers that could be targeted with FGFR inhibitors (8):

- Mutually exclusive with HER2 positivity, that is, FGFR2 alterations are present only in HER2-negative tumors (9).
- In HER2-negative G/GOJ adenocarcinomas, around 30% have been found to have FGFR2 overexpression or *FGFR2* gene amplification (8).
- The phase II FIGHT trial showed benefit of bemarituzumab (FGFR2b selective antibody) compared to placebo combined with first-line FOLFOX6 chemotherapy. The trial included HER2-negative patients with FGFR2b overexpression (any 2+/3+ staining) by centrally performed IHC or FGFR2 amplification by circulating tumor DNA (ctDNA). In the overall trial population, the addition of bemarituzumab to chemotherapy showed an improvement of median OS by 5.7 months (19.2 vs. 13.5 months). In the subgroup of patients with ≥10% FGFR2b+ by IHC, there was doubling of median OS by addition of bemarituzumab—25.4 vs. 11.1 months (8).
- Multiple clinical trials are currently ongoing with various FGFR inhibitors in patients with advanced gastric cancers.

CLDN18.2

Tight junction molecule claudin-18 isoform 2 (CLDN18.2) expression can be assessed on IHC as a predictive biomarker for CLDN18.2-directed therapy (10):

- The phase II FAST trial investigated the addition of zolbetuximab (anti-CLDN18.2 antibody) to first-line EOX (epirubicin, oxaliplatin, capecitabine) chemotherapy. The inclusion criteria based

on CLDN18.2 expression were defined as ≥40% of tumor cells with 2+ or 3+ staining intensity on IHC assay, which was present in around 45% of patient samples screened.
- In the overall population, the addition of zolbetuximab improved median OS by 4.8 months (13.0 vs. 8.3 months). In the subgroup of patients with >70% of tumor cells positive for CLDN18.2 (70%–74% of study population), the median OS was doubled by the addition of zolbetuximab (16.5 vs. 8.9 months) (10).
- Multiple phase III trials are ongoing using CLDN18.2 expression in ≥75% of tumor cells as an inclusion criteria (11).

MSI and TMB

MSI and tumor mutational burden (TMB) have become tumor-agnostic predictive biomarkers for immunotherapy. Similarly, in upper gastrointestinal cancers, a small percentage of MSI-high and TMB-high cancers have been found:

- MSI has been found in around 3% to 4% of patients with advanced gastric/GOJ cancers (12).
- A single-arm trial with pembrolizumab monotherapy in MSI-high non–colorectal patients showed ORR 34.3%; median progression-free survival (PFS) 4.1 months, and median OS 23.5 months (13).
- High TMB has been found in around 12% of advanced gastric cancers (14).
- The Keynote 128 trial investigated single-agent pembrolizumab in various cancer types and showed that in the subgroup of patients with high TMB defined as ≥10 mutations per megabase (13% of all tumor types), the ORR was 29%, compared to 6% in the TMB-low subgroup (15). However, this trial did not include patients with upper gastrointestinal cancers.

DDR Mutations

DNA damage repair (DDR)- and homologous recombination deficiency (HRD)-related mutations have been found in various cancers and have become predictive biomarkers for poly (ADP-ribose) polymerase (PARP) inhibitor—and platinum sensitivity. Although PARP inhibitor responses have been clearest in germline breast cancer (BRCA)1/2 mutated tumors, somatic BRCA mutations and other DDR alterations have similarly shown sensitivity to PARP inhibition.

- In G/GOJ cancers, germline DDR mutations are rare and present in around 1% to 2% of patients, whereas wider DDR/HRD mutations like PALB2, ATM, ARID1A, and others have been found in 10% to 15% of patients (16).
- Olaparib (PARP inhibitor) was investigated in the placebo-controlled phase III GOLD clinical trial where it was added to standard second-line paclitaxel treatment (unselected patients). This trial failed to show statistically significant difference between olaparib and placebo when added to paclitaxel in all patients and even in the prespecified subgroups with HRD or ATM loss (17).
- Currently the role of DDR/HRD-related mutations in G/GOJ cancers is unknown, but various other trials are currently ongoing with PARP inhibitors (18–20).

Other Rare Alterations

In addition to more common alterations, around 1% of patients with G/GOJ cancer also harbor alterations in other potentially targetable genes like $KRAS^{G12C}$, $BRAF^{V600E}$, and NTRK (fusion). Recent basket trials including various tumor types with these alterations have shown promising results. For example, as one of the first tumor-agnostic targets, NTRK fusions have become part of standard next-generation sequencing (NGS) testing for all cancers because of the very promising response rates with TRK inhibitors. Several trials with $KRAS^{G12C}$ inhibitors are currently ongoing and including also upper gastrointestinal tract tumors.

Actionable Target	Abnormality	Prevalence (%)	Clinical Experience with Targeted Agent
HER2	Overexpression/ amplification	22 gastric/ gastroesophageal junction, adenocarcinoma (21)	**Trastuzumab (HER2 inhibitor):** Phase III trial with cisplatin, 5-FU, or capecitabine: median OS 13.8 vs. 11.1 months (2) **Trastuzumab deruxtecan (HER2 antibody–drug conjugate with a topoisomerase I inhibitor):** Third line or beyond—Phase II trial trastuzumab deruxtecan vs. chemotherapy: ORR 51% vs. 14%; OS 12.5 vs. 8.4 months, respectively (3)
PD-L1	PD-L1 CPS ≥10	49.9–52.4 (Keynote 590) esophageal/ gastroesophageal junction, adenocarcinoma/squamous cell carcinoma (4)	**Esophageal** **Pembrolizumab (PD-1 antibody):** First line: Phase III Keynote 590: cisplatin, 5-FU, and pembrolizumab/placebo—median OS all patients 12.4 vs. 9.8, ESCC[+] CPS ≥ 10 = 13.9 vs. 8.8 months (4)
	Tumor cell PD-L1 ≥1%	48.8 (Checkmate 648) esophageal, squamous cell carcinoma (5)	**Nivolumab (anti-PD-1):** First-line CheckMate 648 (squamous cell carcinoma only): Nivolumab and chemotherapy (fluorouracil + cisplatin) or nivolumab + ipilimumab or chemotherapy alone: median OS in PD-L1 ≥ 1–15.4 vs. 13.7 vs. 9.1 months, respectively. OS in all patients 13.2 vs. 12.8 vs. 10.7 months, respectively (5)

Actionable Target	Abnormality	Prevalence (%)	Clinical Experience with Targeted Agent
	PD-L1 CPS ≥5	62 (Checkmate 649) gastric/gastroesophageal junction/esophageal, adenocarcinoma (6)	**Gastric** **Nivolumab (anti-PD-1):** Phase III trial Checkmate 649 (gastric/gastroesophageal junction/esophageal adenocarcinoma): doublet chemotherapy and nivolumab/placebo. Median OS in CPS ≥5= 14.4 vs. 11.1 months and OS in all patients 13.8 vs. 11.6 months, respectively (6)
FGFR	FGFR2b overexpression *FGFR2* gene amplification	30.2 (of HER2 negative) gastric/gastroesophageal junction, adenocarcinoma (8)	**Bemarituzumab (FGFR2b selective antibody):** Phase II trial FOLFOX6 + bemarituzumab or placebo: OS 19.2 vs. 13.5 months; in patients with ≥10% FGFR2b+ (by IHC)— OS 25.4 vs. 11.1 months (8)
Claudin 18.2	Moderate to strong CLDN18.2 expression in >70% of tumor cells	32.4 gastric/gastroesophageal junction, adenocarcinoma (10)	**Zolbetuximab (anti-CLDN18.2 antibody):** Phase II trial EOX + zolbetuximab or EOX alone: OS 13.0 vs. 8.3 months in the whole population; 16.5 vs. 8.9 months in patients with >70% of tumor cells positive for CLDN18.2 (10)

(*continued*)

Actionable Target	Abnormality	Prevalence (%)	Clinical Experience with Targeted Agent
MSI	MSI-High	<2% esophageal, squamous cell carcinoma ~15% gastric, adenocarcinoma (12)	**Pembrolizumab (PD-1 antibody):** Phase II single-arm trial with monotherapy in MSI-high patients: ORR 34.3%; median PFS 4.1 months and median OS 23.5 months (13)
TMB	High ≥10 mutations/megabase	13 gastric, adenocarcinoma (14)	**Pembrolizumab (PD-1 antibody):** Phase II open-label trial of pembrolizumab monotherapy. ORR in TMB-high 29% vs. nonhigh 6% (15)
DNA damage repair (DDR) mutations	HRD mutations: BRCA1/2 PALB2 ATM ARID1A and others	10–15 gastric/gastroesophageal junction, adenocarcinoma (16,17)	**Olaparib (PARP inhibitor):** Negative study: Phase III trial of paclitaxel + olaparib or placebo: OS 8.8 vs. 6.9 months (not statistically significant) (18) Various other trials currently ongoing with olaparib (19,20,22)
KRAS	G12C mutation	0.6 gastric, adenocarcinoma 0.3 esophageal, squamous cell carcinoma (23)	**Sotorasib (KRAS G12C inhibitor):** Phase I trial, ORR 7% (1/15) in various GI cancers (24)

Actionable Target	Abnormality	Prevalence (%)	Clinical Experience with Targeted Agent
BRAF	V600E mutation	0.4 gastric, adeno-carcinoma (25)	**Vemurafenib (BRAF inhibitor):** Phase II basket trial with various BRAF V600E mutant nonmelanoma cancers (including esophageal): ORR 33%, median duration of response 13 months (26)
NTRK	Fusion	0.16 gastric 0.24 esophageal (27,28)	**Entrectinib (TRK inhibitor):** Combination of three, ongoing phase I or II clinical trials of various cancers with NTRK gene fusions: ORR 57%; median duration of response 10 months (27) **Larotrectinib (TRK inhibitor):** Combination of three phase I–II trials: overall response rate was 75%, median duration of response not reached (29)

5-FU, 5-fluorouracil; ARID1A, AT-rich interaction domain 1A; ATM, ataxia telangiectasia mutated; BRAF, B-Raf proto-oncogene; BRCA1/2, breast cancer 1/2; CPS, combined positive score; ESCC, esophageal squamous cell carcinoma; FGFR2, fibroblast growth factor receptor 2; GI, gastrointestinal; HER2, human epidermal growth factor receptor 2; HRD, homologous recombination deficiency; IHC, immunohistochemistry; KRAS, KRAS proto-oncogene; MSI, microsatellite instability; NTRK, neurotrophic receptor tyrosine kinase; ORR, overall response rate; OS, overall survival; PALB2, partner and Localizer of BRCA2; PARP, poly (ADP-ribose) polymerase; PD-L1, programmed death-ligand 1; PFS, progression-free survival; TMB, tumor mutational burden.

CHAPTER 3

Liver Cancer (Hepatocellular)

Irene S. Yu and Ahmed O. Kaseb

Introduction

An estimated 42,230 new cases of liver cancer are diagnosed in the United States annually, with the majority comprised of hepatocellular carcinoma (HCC) cases (1). Five-year overall survival (OS) remains poor at 20% (1). Up until recently, there was a significant unmet need for therapeutic strategies for a disease that was traditionally limited in systemic options, once locoregional treatments have been exhausted. HCC is notably a chemorefractory tumor group and until 2008, there was no standard of care systemic therapy. Historically, systemic chemotherapy regimens included various combinations of gemcitabine, cisplatin, fluoropyrimidine, and/or doxorubicin-based treatments with modest response rates (2–5). Advances in understanding the mechanisms driving tumorigenesis in HCC as well as progress in drug development have led to multiple approvals for immune checkpoint inhibitors and targeted therapies in recent years, and significant evolution in the treatment landscape of advanced HCC.

Vascular Endothelial Growth Factor Pathway

Sorafenib is an oral multikinase inhibitor that targets intracellular Raf kinases and cell surface kinase receptors including vascular endothelial growth factor receptors (VEGFRs)1, 2, and 3, which are implicated in the pathogenesis of HCC (6,7). The phase III SHARP trial led to the U.S. Food and Drug Administration (FDA) approval of sorafenib, which showed a survival benefit of 2.8 months vs. placebo in patients with advanced HCC who did not receive prior systemic therapy (hazard ratio [HR] 0.69, median OS [mOS] 10.7 vs. 7.9 months) (8). Lenvatinib is another oral multikinase inhibitor; its targets include VEGFR1, 2, and 3, fibroblast growth factor receptors (FGFRs)1, 2, 3, 4, and 5, platelet-derived growth factor receptor (PDGFR)-α, KIT, and RET. Lenvatinib emerged as an alternative first-line therapy as it demonstrated noninferiority to sorafenib in the REFLECT trial (HR 0.92, mOS 13.6 vs. 12.3 months), although ORRs were significantly higher at 24.1% vs. 9.2% favoring lenvatinib (9).

Subsequently, several phase III trials in the second-line setting involving regorafenib, ramucirumab, and cabozantinib showed significant OS benefit compared to best supportive care or placebo. Regorafenib is an oral multikinase inhibitor against VEGFR1, 2, and 3, KIT, PDGFR-α, PDGFR-β, FGFR1 and 2, among other targets. The RESORCE trial included patients who progressed on sorafenib and excluded those with intolerance; the use of regorafenib was associated with improved OS compared to placebo (HR 0.63, mOS 10.6 vs. 7.8 months) (10). Ramucirumab is an intravenous recombinant monoclonal antibody that specifically inhibits VEGFR2. It was initially studied in the REACH trial, which did not show an OS benefit compared to best supportive care alone in the second-line setting (11). An unplanned subgroup analysis showed that those patients with α-fetoprotein (AFP) levels of ≥400 ng/mL may have derived benefit; thus, the REACH-2 trial was conducted. In patients with elevated AFP levels, ramucirumab was associated with improved survival (HR 0.71, mOS 8.5 vs. 7.3 months) (12). Thus, the approval for ramucirumab is restricted to those with AFP levels of ≥400 ng/ml.

There have been other agents that have shown promising activity, although not approved in the United States at this time or as a single agent for advanced HCC. Bevacizumab is a recombinant humanized monoclonal antibody against vascular endothelial growth factor (VEGF), which has been shown to have single-agent activity with ORR of 14% in a phase II trial (13). Apatinib is an oral VEGFR2 inhibitor, studied in a phase III study after progression on sorafenib- and oxaliplatin-based chemotherapy. It is associated with OS benefit compared to placebo (HR 0.79, mOS 8.7 vs. 6.8 months) (14). At this time, it is available in China and not in the United States.

MET Overexpression

Cabozantinib was studied in the second-line setting and beyond in the phase III CELESTIAL trial. It is another oral multikinase inhibitor targeting VEGFR1, 2, and 3, but also includes MET, AXL, FLT-3, KIT, RET, and ROS1. In several studies, MET overexpression has been associated with the development of resistance to sorafenib (15,16), thus cabozantinib was studied in the post-sorafenib setting given its activity against MET. Its use was associated with improved OS (HR 0.76, mOS 10.2 vs. 8.0 months) compared to placebo (17) and is indicated as second-line therapy in those previously treated with sorafenib or lenvatinib.

Immune Checkpoint Inhibition

HCC is considered an immunogenic cancer as it often arises from chronic inflammatory conditions (18). As the liver is exposed to many antigens as a part of its normal physiologic function, there is development of intrinsic tolerance in the innate and adaptive immune responses (19). With chronic inflammation, immune suppression contributes to carcinogenesis and thus presents an opportunity for intervention with immunotherapy. There have been ongoing efforts evaluating immune checkpoint inhibitors, initially in the second-line setting and subsequently in the first-line setting both in combination with anti-VEGF therapy or tyrosine kinase inhibitors and as monotherapy.

Nivolumab and Combination Nivolumab/Ipilimumab

CheckMate 040 is a multicohort phase I/II study evaluating the role of nivolumab (PD-1 inhibitor) in advanced HCC. El-Khoueiry et al. evaluated a 3+3 dose escalation cohort followed by an expansion cohort at a dose of 3 mg/kg, in patients with Child Pugh B score of 7 or less (20); ORR was 15% and 20% for the dose escalation and expansion cohorts, respectively. This resulted in the accelerated FDA approval of single-agent nivolumab for the treatment of HCC patients previously treated with sorafenib, but this indication for nivolumab has been withdrawn in 2021, reflecting the results of the CheckMate 459 study. CheckMate 459 was a phase III trial comparing nivolumab and sorafenib in the first-line setting, and did not show a statistically significant OS benefit (HR 0.84, mOS 16.4 vs. 14.7 months) (21).

In a separate cohort of CheckMate 040, Yau et al. randomized patients to three different arms with different dosing of nivolumab and ipilimumab (cytotoxic T-cell lymphocyte antigen-4 [CTLA-4] inhibitor): (i) nivolumab 1 mg/kg + ipilimumab 3 mg/kg every 3 weeks for four doses followed by nivolumab 240 mg every 2 weeks maintenance (arm A), (ii) nivolumab 3 mg/kg + ipilimumab 1 mg/kg every 3 weeks for four doses followed by nivolumab 240 mg every 2 weeks maintenance (arm B), and (iii) nivolumab 3 mg/kg every 2 weeks + ipilimumab 1 mg/kg every 6 weeks ongoing (arm C) (22). Arm A had the highest ORR at 32%, compared to 31% in arm B, and 31% in arm C (23). The arm A combination with nivolumab 1 mg/kg + ipilimumab 3 mg/kg followed by maintenance nivolumab was approved by the FDA in 2020, for those patients previously treated with sorafenib.

Pembrolizumab

Data for pembrolizumab (PD-1 inhibitor) in the post-sorafenib setting were first studied in the phase II KEYNOTE-224 trial, where ORR of 17% was achieved (24). Subsequently, the phase III KEYNOTE-240 trial comparing pembrolizumab to best supportive care did not meet both coprimary endpoints of OS and progression-free survival (PFS) (25). More recently, results from KEYNOTE-394 were reported; this was a phase III study that enrolled Asian patients with advanced HCC who were previously treated with sorafenib or oxaliplatin-based chemotherapy. A significant OS benefit was observed for pembrolizumab compared to placebo (HR 0.79, mOS 14.6 vs. 13.0 months), in addition to a statistically significant but modest PFS benefit (HR 0.74, mPFS 2.6 vs. 2.3 months) (26). The authors also presented a meta-analysis of OS based on data derived from KEYNOTE-394 and KEYNOTE-240; with the pooled data, mOS was 14.2 months compared to 12.5 months (HR 0.79), favoring pembrolizumab (26). Finally, in cohort 2 of KEYNOTE-224, pembrolizumab was evaluated in the first-line setting. Preliminary results presented at ASCO Gastrointestinal Symposium 2021 showed ORR of 16% and median OS of 17 months (27).

Combination Atezolizumab and Bevacizumab

The phase III IMbrave150 trial is a first-line study that compared atezolizumab (PD-L1 inhibitor) + bevacizumab given every 3 weeks against the previous standard of care, sorafenib (28,29). Updated survival data demonstrated improvements in both median OS and PFS favoring atezolizumab/bevacizumab (HR 0.66, mOS 19.2 vs. 13.4 months; HR 0.59, mPFS 6.8 vs. 4.3 months) (28,29). ORR was also improved at 29.8% for atezolizumab/bevacizumab and 11.3% for sorafenib (29). This is currently the standard of care first-line therapy for patients with HCC, if they are eligible for the combination.

Combination Atezolizumab and Cabozantinib

COSMIC-312 is another first-line phase III study; patients were randomized to combination atezolizumab and cabozantinib, sorafenib, and cabozantinib monotherapy (30). Atezolizumab and cabozantinib combination was associated with improved PFS compared to sorafenib (HR 0.63, mPFS 6.8 vs. 4.2 months); however, a statistically significant improvement in OS was not observed at the interim analysis.

Durvalumab and Combination Durvalumab/Tremelimumab

Following the promising results of the phase I/II study of durvalumab (PD-L1 inhibitor) and tremelimumab (CTLA-4 inhibitor) in patients who have progressed, were intolerant of, or refused sorafenib (31), the combination was evaluated in the phase III HIMALAYA trial in the first-line setting. The study encompassed multiple arms, and the STRIDE regimen arm consisting of a single priming dose of tremelimumab 300 mg and durvalumab 1,500 mg every 4 weeks was associated with superior OS compared to sorafenib (HR 0.78, mOS 16.4 vs. 13.8 months) (32). A secondary objective compared durvalumab monotherapy to sorafenib, which met the noninferiority endpoint (HR 0.86, mOS 16.6 vs. 13.8 months) and presents as an immunotherapy as a monotherapy option in the first-line setting (32).

Other Immune Checkpoint Inhibitors

Avelumab is a PD-L1 inhibitor studied in a single-arm phase II study in the post-sorafenib setting. It was associated with ORR of 10% and mOS of 14.2 months (33). Sintilimab is a PD-1 inhibitor available in China, and it has been studied in combination with bevacizumab biosimilar in a phase II/III study compared to sorafenib in the first-line setting, specifically in patients with hepatitis B–associated unresectable HCC. Median PFS was significantly longer (HR 0.56, mPFS 4.6 vs. 2.8 months) compared to sorafenib (34). In the first interim analysis of OS, this also favored sintilimab–bevacizumab biosimilar (HR 0.57, mOS not reached vs. 10.4 months) (35).

PI3K/AKT/mTOR Pathway

The PI3K/AKT/mTOR pathway can be dysregulated frequently in HCC (31). Temsirolimus inhibits mechanistic target of rapamycin (mTOR) by binding to the protein FKBP-12 to form a complex that inhibits mTOR signaling, leading to cell cycle arrest at the G1 phase. In a phase I/II study, temsirolimus was shown to have limited activity with ORR of 3% (36). Everolimus was studied in the phase III EVOLVE-1 study in patients who progressed or were intolerant to sorafenib, and did not improve OS (HR 1.05, mOS 7.6 vs. 7.3 months) (37). At this time, both agents do not play a significant role in the overall treatment of advanced HCC.

Tumor Growth Factor-β Inhibition

Tumor growth factor (TGF)-β is a cytokine that promotes tumorigenesis via its role in epithelial–mesenchymal transition and neoangiogenesis (38,39). Galunisertib is a small-molecule inhibitor of TGF-β1. In a phase II study in the post-sorafenib setting, treatment with galunisertib was associated with ORR of 7.5% and OS of 16.8 months for those patients with AFP levels <1.5 times the upper limit of normal (40). Lower AFP levels were associated with better outcomes, as the ORR was 0% for those patients with AFP ≥1.5 times the upper limit of normal. This has also been studied in combination with sorafenib in another phase II study, and the combination showed mOS of 18.8 months and ORR of 4.5% (41). At this time, galunisertib is not approved but is undergoing further investigation in combination with nivolumab (NCT02423343).

Future Directions

The treatment landscape of advanced HCC is now comprised of immunotherapy and targeted therapy in both first-line and subsequent lines of therapy, with a diminishing role for cytotoxic chemotherapy. Furthermore, there are multiple phase III first-line combinations that are currently being evaluated at this time, including: lenvatinib and pembrolizumab (LEAP-002, NCT03713593), nivolumab and ipilimumab (CheckMate 9DW, NCT04039607), and tislelizumab (PD-1 inhibitor, RATIONALE-301, NCT03412773). A pivotal area of unmet need will be determining the optimal sequence of therapy after first-line combination therapies and this will become even more important if additional upcoming first-line studies show a positive outcome in OS.

Actionable Target	Abnormality	Prevalence (%)	Clinical Experience with Targeted Agent
VEGF	Overexpression	77	**Regorafenib** (multikinase inhibitor): • Phase III: ORR 11% vs. 4%, PFS 3.1 vs. 1.5 months, OS 10.6 vs. 7.8 months compared to placebo, *2L post-sorafenib* (10) **Ramucirumab** (anti-VEGF): • Phase III: ORR 5% vs. 1%, PFS 2.8 vs. 1.6 months, OS 8.5 vs. 7.3 months compared to placebo, *2L post-sorafenib and AFP ≥ 400 ng/mL* (12) **Bevacizumab** (anti-VEGF): • Phase II: ORR 14%, PFS 3 months, OS 8 months, *1L or 2L* (13) **Apatinib** (anti-VEGF): • Phase III: ORR 11% vs. 2%, PFS 4.5 vs. 1.9 months, OS 8.7 vs. 6.8 months compared to placebo, *2L+* (14)
MET	Overexpression	70	**Cabozantinib** (multikinase inhibitor): • Phase III: ORR 4% vs. <1%, PFS 5.2 vs. 1.9 months, OS 10.2 vs. 8.0 months compared to placebo, *2L+ post-sorafenib* (17)
PD-L1	Overexpression	27	**Nivolumab** (anti-PD-1): • Phase III: ORR 15% vs. 7%, PFS 3.7 vs. 3.8 months[NS], OS 16.4 vs. 14.7 months[NS] compared to sorafenib, *1L* (21)

(continued)

Actionable Target	Abnormality	Prevalence (%)	Clinical Experience with Targeted Agent
			• Phase I/II: ORR 20%, PFS 4 months, OS NR, 6 months OS 83% for dose-expansion cohort, *1L+* (20)
			Nivolumab + ipilimumab (anti-CTLA-4): • Phase I/II: ORR 32%, OS 22.2 months for nivolumab 1 mg/kg + ipilimumab 3 mg/kg × 4 cycles → nivolumab 240 mg q2w, *2L+ post-sorafenib* (22,23)
			Pembrolizumab (anti-PD-1): • Phase II: ORR 16%, PFS 4 months, OS 17 months, *1L* (27) • Phase II: ORR 17%, PFS 4.9 months, OS 12.9 months, *2L post-sorafenib* (24) • Phase III: ORR 18.3% vs. 4.4%, PFS 3.0 vs. 2.8 months, OS 13.9 vs. 10.6 months compared to placebo, *2L post-sorafenib* (25) • Phase III: ORR 12.7% vs. 1.3%, PFS 2.6 vs. 2.3 months, OS 14.6 vs. 13.0 months compared to placebo, *2L post-sorafenib or oxaliplatin-based chemotherapy* (26)
			Bevacizumab + atezolizumab (anti-PD-L1): • Phase III: ORR 29.8% vs. 11.3%, PFS 6.8 vs. 4.3 months, OS 19.2 vs. 13.4 months compared to sorafenib, *1L* (28,29)

Actionable Target	Abnormality	Prevalence (%)	Clinical Experience with Targeted Agent
			Cabozantinib + atezolizumab: • Phase III: ORR 11% vs. 3.7%, PFS 6.8 vs. 4.2 months, OS 15.4 vs. 15.5 months[NS] compared to sorafenib, *1L* (30)
			Durvalumab (anti-PD-L1): • Phase III: ORR 17.0% vs. 5.1%, PFS 3.65 vs. 4.07 months[NS], OS 16.6 vs. 13.8 months compared to sorafenib[NI], *1L* (32)
			Durvalumab + tremelimumab (anti-CTLA-4): • Phase II: ORR 24%, OS 18.7 months for STRIDE regimen, *1L+* (31) • Phase III: ORR 20.1% vs. 5.1%, PFS 3.78 vs. 4.07 months[NS], OS 16.4 vs. 13.8 months compared to sorafenib, *1L* (32)
			Avelumab (anti-PD-L1): • Phase II: ORR 10%, PFS 3.5 months, OS 14.2 months, *2L+ post-sorafenib* (33)
			Sintilimab (anti-PD-1) + **bevacizumab:** • Phase II/III: ORR 21% vs. 4%, PFS 4.6 vs. 2.8 months, OS NR vs. 10.4 months compared to sorafenib, *1L* (34) • Sintilimab not available in the United States, only in China

(*continued*)

Actionable Target	Abnormality	Prevalence (%)	Clinical Experience with Targeted Agent
PIK3CA	Mutation	28–36	**Everolimus** (mTOR inhibitor): • Phase III: ORR 2.2% vs. 1.6%, PFS 3.0 vs. 2.6 months[NS], OS 7.6 vs. 7.3 months[NS] compared to placebo, *2L post-sorafenib* (37)
TSC1/2	Mutation	16	
PTEN	Mutation	5	**Temsirolimus** (mTOR inhibitor): • Phase I/II: ORR 3%, PFS 2.8 months, OS 8.9 months, *1L+* (36)
TGF-β	Overexpression	84	**Galunisertib** (TGF-β1): • Phase II: ORR 0/7.5%, PFS 2.7/4.2 months, OS 7.3/16.8 months for AFP ≥ 1.5× ULN/<1.5× ULN, *2L post-sorafenib* (40) **Galunisertib + sorafenib:** • Phase II: ORR 4.5%, PFS 4.1 months, OS 18.8 months for galunisertib 150 mg BID dosing, *1L* (41)

1L, first line; 1L+, first line and beyond; 2L, second line; 2L, second line and beyond; AFP, α-fetoprotein; BID, twice-daily; CTLA-4, cytotoxic T-cell lymphocyte antigen-4; NI, noninferior; NR, not reached; NS, nonsignificant; ORR, overall response rate; OS, overall survival; PD-L1, programmed death ligand 1; PFS, progression-free survival; TGF, tumor growth factor; ULN, upper limit of normal; VEGF, vascular endothelial growth factor.

CHAPTER 4

Biliary Tract Cancer

Sunyoung S. Lee and Milind Javle

Molecular Targeted Therapy

- The molecular analyses of molecular profiling show that up to 35% of patients with cholangiocarcinoma have potentially targetable genomic alterations (1).
- Gene mutations commonly found in cholangiocarcinoma are categorized into five subgroups: receptor tyrosine kinases (FGFR), cell cycle–related genes (TP53, CDKN2A mutation/deletion, and CCND1 amplification), IDH1/2 alterations, MAPK pathway (KRAS, NRAS, and BRAF), and chromatin modifying (ARID1A/B, BAP1, and PBRM1) (2–4).
- Patients with FGFR2 alterations show better prognosis, and those with KRAS and TP53 mutations have worse prognosis. IDH1/2 alterations are neutral in prognosis. BAP1 is related to a more aggressive subtype and associated with poor prognosis.

IDH1 MUTATION

- Isocitrate dehydrogenase (IDH) mutations (IDH1 and 2) are found in 20% to 25% of patients with intrahepatic cholangiocarcinoma.
- An IDH1 inhibitor, ivosidenib (ClarIDHy trial) showed a modest survival benefit (5). Patients who progressed on placebo crossed over to ivosidenib: ORR, 2%; DCR, 53%; mPFS, 2.7 months. In an earlier analysis, 32% and 22% of patients on ivosidenib did not progress at 6 and 12 months (6).
- Ivosidenib was recently approved by the FDA in the second-line setting.

FGFR2 GENE ALTERATIONS

- Fibroblast growth factor receptor 2 (FGFR2) alterations are commonly found in 14% to 20% of patients with intrahepatic cholangiocarcinoma (7,8).
- Pemigatinib, an FDA-approved inhibitor of FGFR1, 2, and 3, showed ORR, DCR, and median duration of response (mDOR) of 35.5%, 80.0%, and 7.5 months in FGFR2 fusions/rearrangements. Patients with other FGFR alterations or no FGF/FGFR alterations showed stable disease in 40% and 22% patients with no overall response.

- Infigratinib, another FDA-approved inhibitor of FGFR1, 2, and 3, showed ORR of 23.1% (35% in the second-line setting and 13.8% in the third- and later-line settings) in FGFR2 fusions or rearrangements; mPFS, 7.3 months (9).
- Futibatinib, an inhibitor of FGFR1, 2, 3, and 4 (10,11), showed mDOR of 6.2 months, ORR of 34.3%, and DCR of 76.1%.
- Common adverse events from FGFR inhibitors include hyperphosphatemia, arthralgias, and ophthalmologic side effects including serous retinal detachment and dry eyes.

ERBB2 (HER2) AMPLIFICATION

- HER2 (ERBB2) amplification is found in intrahepatic (3%), hilar and distal cholangiocarcinoma (11%), and gallbladder carcinoma (16%) (12). The role or sequence of HER2 blockade has not been established.
- A phase II trial of trastuzumab and pertuzumab with 39 patients with HER2 amplification, HER2 overexpression, or both showed ORR and DCR of 23% and 51%, respectively; mDOR, 10.8 months; mPFS and mOS of 4.0 and 10.9 months, respectively (13).
- A phase II, randomized trial of capecitabine with varlitinib, an inhibitor of HER1 (EGFR), HER2, and HER4 in the second-line setting, was recently reported in advanced biliary tract cancer (14). This study did not meet its primary endpoints of ORR and PFS as they were not statistically significantly different. An exploratory analysis showed a trend toward an improved median PFS in female patients and those with gallbladder carcinoma.
- A retrospective study of 14 patients with HER2-amplified biliary tract cancers revealed one complete response, four partial responses, and three stable disease achieved by lapatinib, pertuzumab, or trastuzumab (15).
- Multiple clinical trials are ongoing, and these will be reported in the near future.

BRAF V600

- BRAF V600 mutations are found in 1% to 5% of biliary tract cancer, and it is more commonly found in intrahepatic cholangiocarcinoma (16,17).

- A phase II trial of dabrafenib and trametinib, combination of BRAF and MEK inhibitors in BRAF V600E-mutated biliary tract cancer, showed the ORR and DCR of 47% and 61%; mOS and mPFS, 14 and 9 months, respectively (18).

Immune Checkpoint Blockade

- Data on immunotherapy are still emerging with mixed results, and its role in biliary tract cancer is not well established.
- The percentage of tumors with microsatellite instability (MSI) or mismatch repair deficiency (dMMR) is low and ranges from 1% to 10% in biliary tract cancer (19–21).
- Biliary tract cancer with MSI or dMMR, overexpression of programmed death 1 ligand 1 (PD-L1), and high tumor mutational burden (TMB) may show better response from immunotherapy (22).
- A phase II trial (KEYNOTE-158) with 22 patients having dMMR cholangiocarcinoma showed 41% of ORR, and mDOR from 4.1 to 24.9 months.
- A combined analysis of KEYNOTE-028 and 158 trials suggests that pembrolizumab may have limited activity in cholangiocarcinoma, regardless of PD-L1 expression (23).
- Out of 42 patients who enrolled in a phase II trial of nivolumab, 18 patients (43%) had PD-L1 overexpression, and 10 patients all of whom are with prominent MMR showed partial response. Four out of 10 patients had response that lasted over 1 year (24). This suggests that PD-L1 overexpression is more frequently seen in responders, whereas PD-L1-negative tumors may also respond.
- A phase II trial of nivolumab and ipilimumab or gemcitabine and cisplatin with addition of nivolumab showed inferior PFS from nivolumab + ipilimumab; gemcitabine, cisplatin, and nivolumab are not superior to gemcitabine and cisplatin (25).
- A recent phase III trial (TOPAZ-1) of the addition of an anti-PD-1, durvalumab, to first-line chemotherapy showed clinically meaningful OS benefit vs. chemotherapy alone. This combination also demonstrated an improvement in PFS and ORR (26). Patients received 1,500 mg of durvalumab every 3 weeks with 1,000 mg/m^2 of gemcitabine and 25 mg/m^2 of cisplatin on days 1 and 8 and then every 3 weeks up to eight cycles, followed by durvalumab 1,500 mg every four

cycles or placebo until disease progression or unacceptable toxicity. Primary endpoint was OS; secondary endpoints were progression-free survival (PFS), ORR and safety. Results showed the following:

- At data cutoff for the interim analysis (August 11, 2021), the durvalumab group had improved OS with a hazard ratio (HR) of 0.80 (95% confidence interval [CI], 0.66–0.97; $p = 0.021$).
- PFS was significantly improved for the durvalumab group (HR 0.75; 95% CI, 0.64–0.89; $p = 0.001$). ORR was 26.7% for durvalumab and 18.7% for placebo. Grade 3 or 4 treatment-related adverse events were seen in 62.7% of durvalumab patients and 64.9% of those taking placebo.
- Patients having solid tumors with high TMB may benefit from immunotherapy in various tumor types (27,28). Pembrolizumab is approved by the FDA for tumor types with a TMB ≥ 10 mutations/megabase (29).
- Assessment of mutational profiles, PD-L1 expression, and TMB is of essence in treating patients with advanced or metastatic biliary tract cancer.
- Combination of pembrolizumab and lenvatinib (inhibitor of VEGFR1, 2, and 3, FGFR1, 2, 3, and 4, and platelet-derived growth factor receptor α, KIT, and RET) in biliary tract cancer (BTC) ($N = 31$) showed ORR of 10%, DCR of 21%, and median DOR of 5.3 months (30). It is recommended by NCCN as of September 2021.

Key actionable mutations in cholangiocarcinoma with clinical data

Actionable Target	Abnormality	Prevalence (%)	Clinical Experience with Targeted Agent
IDH1	Somatic	20–25	Intrahepatic cholangiocarcinoma Ivosidenib (IDH1 inhibition, ClarIDHy) • Phase III: ORR 2%, DCR 53%, PFS 2.7 months
FGFR2 fusion	Somatic, fusion	14–20	Mainly intrahepatic cholangiocarcinoma Pemigatinib (FGFR inhibition) • Phase II: ORR 35.5%, DCR 80%, DOR 7.5 months • Other FGFR alteration: SD 40% • No FGF/FGFR alterations: SD 22% Infigratinib (FGFR inhibition) • Phase II: ORR 23.1%, PFS 7.3 months Futibatinib (FGFR inhibition) • Phase II: ORR 34.3%, DCR 76.1%, DOR 6.2 months
HER2 amplification	Somatic, amplification	3–16	Trastuzumab and pertuzumab (39 pts) • Phase II: ORR 23%, DCR 51%, DOR 10.8 months • OS and PFS, 10.9 and 4.0 months

Actionable Target	Abnormality	Prevalence (%)	Clinical Experience with Targeted Agent
BRAF V600	Somatic	1–5	More common in intrahepatic cholangiocarcinoma Dabrafenib and trametinib • Phase II: ORR 47%, DCR 61% • OS and PFS, 14 and 9 months
MSI-High	MSI-High	1–10	Pembrolizumab (KEYNOTE-158, 22 pts) • Phase II: ORR 41%, DOR 4.1-24.9 months
PD-L1 overexpression		43	Pembrolizumab Out of 42 pts, 18 pts (43%) • Phase II: ORR (10/18) • PD-L1 negative tumors may respond
TMB ≥ 10/Mb		Varies	Pembrolizumab approved for any solid tumors in this clinical scenario (Phase II)

DCR, disease control rate; DOR, duration of response; FGF, fibroblast growth factor; FGFR, fibroblast growth factor receptor; MSI, microsatellite instability; ORR, objective response rate; OS, overall survival; PD-L1, programmed death-ligand 1; PFS, progression-free survival; SD, stable disease; TMB, tumor mutation burden.

CHAPTER 5

Pancreatic Cancer

Michael Sangmin Lee, Tanios Bekaii-Saab, and Shubham Pant

Introduction

Pancreatic cancer is the third most common cancer causing mortality in the United States. Despite improvements in mortality rates observed in many other cancer types in the last 5 to 10 years, the mortality rate from pancreatic cancer has been stable in women and increasing in men at 0.3% per year since 2000 (1). The majority of patients (52%) who are diagnosed with pancreatic cancer have distant metastatic disease at diagnosis (1), and even in patients with resectable disease who are treated with adjuvant chemotherapy, 3-year disease-free survival rate is only 39.7% with adjuvant FOLFIRINOX chemotherapy (2) and 20.9% with adjuvant gemcitabine + capecitabine (3), demonstrating the high risk of recurrence even in patients with earlier stage disease. For patients with metastatic disease, the standard of care first-line chemotherapy regimens include FOLFIRINOX and gemcitabine + nab-paclitaxel, but median overall survival is only 8.5 to 11.1 months (4,5). Until recently, there were no predictive biomarkers to enable selection of patients to receive targeted therapy or immunotherapy. However, with emerging data, national guidelines now recommend testing pancreatic cancer for germline mutations, somatic mutations and fusions, and microsatellite instability/mismatch repair deficiency (6), as results impact both standard of care options and eligibility for promising clinical trials of targeted therapies with compelling preclinical data.

Germline Mutations Impacting DNA Damage Repair Pathways

Multiple studies have shown roughly 4% to 10% of pancreatic cancers harbor deleterious germline mutations (7–11) (Table 5.1), with roughly half of patients with a germline mutation lacking a suspicious family history (9). Given this, consensus guidelines recommend germline testing for all patients with pancreatic adenocarcinoma (12).

1. Germline *BRCA1/2* mutations. Inheritance of one defective *BRCA1/2* allele and loss of heterozygosity of the second allele cause homologous recombination defects (HRDs), causing aberrant DNA damage repair and increasing susceptibility to chemotherapy agents that cause double-stranded DNA breaks, like platinum agents. Indeed, a prospective phase II trial showed gemcitabine + cisplatin backbone had response rate of 70% in HRD metastatic

pancreatic cancer (13), and retrospective data also show improved progression-free survival (PFS) with first-line platinum-based regimen, with most patients receiving FOLFIRINOX (14). The phase III POLO trial found that in patients with germline BRCA1/2 mutations who receive induction platinum-based chemotherapy with disease control after 4 to 6 months, maintenance therapy with the poly (ADP-ribose) polymerase (PARP) inhibitor olaparib significantly improved PFS compared to placebo (median PFS 7.4 vs. 3.8 months, hazard ratio [HR] 0.53, 95% confidence interval [CI] 0.35–0.82) (15). However, maintenance olaparib did not significantly improve OS (HR 0.83, 95% CI 0.56–1.22) (16). Nevertheless, olaparib maintenance therapy is now U.S. Food and Drug Administration (FDA) approved. Additional combinations of DNA damage repair inhibitors and immunotherapy agents are currently in clinical trials.

2. Germline PALB2. PALB2 mutations also confer HRD, similar to BRCA1/2 mutations, and studies, albeit with limited numbers of patients, suggest sensitivity to platinum agents (13) and to PARP inhibitors like rucaparib (17).

3. Germline ATM mutations. Deleterious ATM germline mutations are in 1.7% to 3.3% of pancreatic cancers (18,19). PARP inhibitor monotherapy has shown limited disease control in case reports of germline ATM-mutated pancreatic cancer (20,21), but there are promising data of multiple DNA damage repair (DDR) therapies targeting ATM, ATR, CHK1, or combinations of DDR agents (19,22).

Microsatellite Instability

Microsatellite instability (MSI) is found in 1% to 2% of pancreatic adenocarcinoma, particularly associated with mucinous/colloid and medullary histology (23). Pembrolizumab and dostarlimab-gxly are FDA approved for previously treated MSI cancers given response rate of 34.3% and 41.6%, respectively, among MSI solid tumors (24,25). In an early study of pembrolizumab in MSI cancers, 5/8 (62%) pancreatic cancers had a response, including 2 (25%) complete responses (26). In the small 22-patient pancreatic cancer cohort of KEYNOTE-158, pembrolizumab treatment yielded response rate of 18.2% (95% CI 5.2–40.3), with median duration of response 13.4 months (24).

Actionable Target	Abnormality	Prevalence (%)	Clinical Experience with Targeted Agent
BRCA1/2	Germline mutation	3–5	Platinum chemotherapy Maintenance therapy with olaparib (PARP inhibitor) • Median PFS 7.4 months (vs. 3.8 months with placebo) (15) • Median OS 19.0 months (vs. 19.2 months with placebo) (16)
PALB2	Germline mutation	0.6	Platinum chemotherapy Rucaparib: 2/2 patients had response (17).
ATM	Germline mutation	1.7–3.3	Case reports suggest resistance to PARP inhibitor (20,21).
MSI-High	MSI-High	1–2	Pembrolizumab (KEYNOTE-158) • 5/8 (62%) pancreatic cancer patients in a phase II study had CR or PR (26). • Of 22 pancreatic cancer patients, ORR 18.2%, median DOR 13.4 months (24) Dostarlimab (GARNET) • Of four pancreatic cancer patients, one SD and three PD (25)
KRAS G12C	Mutation	1	Sotorasib (AMG510) • 1/11 PR, 8/11 SD, 2/11 PD (27) Adagrasib (MRTX849) • One patient with confirmed response (28)

CR, complete response; DOR, duration of response; ORR, overall response rate; OS, overall survival; PARP, poly (ADP-ribose) polymerase; PD, progressive disease; PFS, progression-free survival; PR, partial response; SD, stable disease.

KRAS Oncogenic Mutations and Targeting

Oncogenic KRAS mutations occur in 90% to 93% of pancreatic cancers (29,30). KRAS is a small GTPase that cycles between an active GTP-bound state and an inactive GDP-bound state. Activating KRAS mutations cause an increase in active GTP-bound KRAS, activating the RAF-MEK-ERK and other effector pathways to increase proliferation and survival (31). Until recently, there have not been any effective direct inhibitors of KRAS, but insights into the biophysics and biochemistry of KRAS have enabled development of novel promising inhibitors.

1. KRAS G12C. In pancreatic cancer, G12D, G12V, and G12R are the most common mutations in KRAS; G12C mutations are found in 1% of pancreatic cancer (29,30). A new generation of KRAS G12C-specific inhibitors, like sotorasib (AMG510) and adagrasib (MRTX849), can directly bind to and inhibit the mutant protein (32). Single-agent sotorasib or adagrasib has shown cases of partial responses in KRAS G12C mutant pancreatic cancer (27,33), and multiple additional KRAS G12C inhibitors are currently in development. Ongoing clinical trials are assessing the safety and efficacy of novel combinations of G12C inhibitors with RAF-MEK-ERK pathway inhibitors, immune checkpoint inhibitors, and other targeted agents.

2. SHP2 inhibitors. SHP2 is a protein tyrosine phosphatase that is activated by a number of cell surface receptor tyrosine kinases (RTKs) and facilitates KRAS loading with GTP and helps drive feedback reactivation of RAS-RAF-MEK-ERK signaling after MEK inhibitor therapy (34,35). SHP2 inhibitors impaired activation of KRAS codon 12 mutant proteins and synergized with MEK inhibitor and G12C inhibitor in preclinical models (36,37). Multiple clinical trials of SHP2 inhibitors alone or in combination with other targeted drugs like MEK inhibitors or KRAS G12C inhibitors are underway.

3. SOS1 inhibitors. SOS1 is a guanine exchange factor (GEF) that catalyzes GDP–GTP exchange, and attempts to block the RAF-MEK-ERK pathway with MEK inhibitors cause feedback reactivation via SOS1 to promote GTP loading of KRAS (38). Novel small molecule inhibitors that impair SOS1–KRAS binding decreased proliferation in almost all KRAS codon 12 and 13 mutants tested preclinically and synergized with MEK inhibitors (39). Clinical trials of SOS1 inhibitors like BI1701963 alone and combined with MEK inhibitors and KRAS G12C inhibitors are ongoing.

4. Additional KRAS mutation-specific approaches:
   a. Oligonucleotide therapies cause degradation of target mRNA molecules to decrease target gene expression. Oligonucleotide therapies targeting specific KRAS G12D mutant sequences and packaged in optimal drug delivery vehicles like exosomes are now in clinical trials (40).
   b. Mutation-specific immune approaches have been of interest since HLA-restricted T cells recognizing KRAS G12D or KRAS G12V were identified in specific cases (41,42), stoking interest in potential cellular therapies targeting specific mutations. mRNA vaccines targeting the most common KRAS mutations are also in development (43).

Genomic Aberrations Enriched in KRAS Wild-Type Cancers

About 7% to 10% of pancreatic cancers are KRAS wild type (WT) (29), more commonly found in patients under age 50 (44). Up to 38% of KRAS WT tumors have driver mutations or fusions activating the RAS-MAPK pathway (44), most with potential targeted therapies (Table 5.2).

1. BRAF mutations, in-frame deletions, and fusions. A range of aberrations causing constitutive activation of BRAF are described in KRAS WT pancreatic cancers. The most common BRAF mutation is in BRAF V600E, and ongoing studies of BRAF inhibitors +/− MEK inhibitors are ongoing. However, other BRAF point mutations, in-frame deletions, and fusions have heterogeneous effects on kinase activation and dimerization, and various BRAF inhibitors have differing ability to bind to the mutant BRAF protein and effectively prevent dimerization (45–47). Combinations of BRAF and MEK inhibitors or monotherapy with ERK inhibitors are being studied.

2. NRG1 fusions. NRG1 encodes neuregulin, a ligand of ERBB3, which dimerizes with HER2 to activate downstream signaling. Activating in-frame NRG1 fusions with high expression have been found to be enriched in KRAS WT pancreatic cancer (48,49). Case reports have shown responses with ERBB family–directed therapies including afatinib and a bispecific ERBB2/ERBB3 antibody zenocutuzumab (MCLA-128) (50,51).

3. NTRK1/2/3 fusions. The NTRK inhibitors larotrectinib and entrectinib are FDA approved for patients with TRK fusion cancers agnostic of tumor type, and although *NTRK* fusions are rare in pancreatic cancer, responses with these drugs are also observed in pancreatic cancers harboring NTRK fusions (52,53).

Additional Targetable Aberrations

1. Methylthioadenosine phosphorylase (MTAP) deletion. MTAP is codeleted with the tumor suppressor CDKN2A (p16), which is also on chromosome 9p, in 25% of pancreatic cancers. MTAP loss causes accumulation of its substrate and inhibits the activity of protein arginine methyltransferase 5 (PRMT5), causing synergistic lethality with PRMT inhibitors or with inhibitors of methionine adenosyltransferase 2a (MAT2A), which further decreases PRMT5 activity (54,55). Clinical trials of MAT2A inhibitors in MTAP-deleted pancreatic cancer are ongoing.

Actionable Target	Abnormality	% of KRAS WT	Clinical Experience with Targeted Agent
BRAF	Mutation: Most commonly V600E, but includes additional mutations (D594G, G469V, G469S)	3.1	BRAF inhibitor ± MEK inhibitor Case reports or small trials showed PR with vemurafenib (56,57) or improved CA19 with dabrafenib + trametinib (58)
BRAF	Activating in-frame intragenic deletions: Most commonly ΔN486_P490 (ΔNVTAP)	3.6	Specific BRAF inhibitors depending on ability to bind the mutant protein ERK inhibitor Case report showed PR with dabrafenib (59)
BRAF	Fusion: Most commonly SND1-BRAF	3.6	Specific BRAF inhibitors depending on ability to inhibit BRAF dimerization ERK inhibitor One patient on clinical trial had PR with vemurafenib (60)
NRG1	Fusion	5.5–7.5	ERBB family inhibitors 2/3 patients responded to afatinib or erlotinib + pertuzumab (48,50) Zenocutuzumab (MCLA-128): Bispecific HER2/HER3 antibody. ORR 5/12 (42%), DCR 92% (51)

(continued)

Table 5.2: Pancreatic cancer (KRAS wild-type) (*continued*)

Actionable Target	Abnormality	% of KRAS WT	Clinical Experience with Targeted Agent
FGFR1/2/3	Fusion	2.7	FGFR inhibitors (erdafitinib, pemigatinib) Erdafitinib showed PR (61)
RAF1	Fusion	1.6	RAF inhibitors Clinical development of RAF inhibitors is ongoing
ALK	Fusion	1.1	ALK inhibitors (crizotinib, ceritinib, alectinib) 3/4 patients had disease control or response (62)
RET	Fusion	<1	Selpercatinib with 2/2 SD (63) Pralsetinib with 3/3 PRs (64)
MET	Fusion	<1	MET inhibitors (crizotinib) Case report showed CR lasting over 12 months (61)
NTRK1/2/3	Fusion	<1	Entrectinib 2/3 patients had PR (52) Larotrectinib 1/1 patient had PR (53)
HER2	Amplification	3.4	Trastuzumab + pertuzumab ORR was 1/10 (10%) In KRAS WT was 1/3 (33.3%) (65)

Note: KRAS WT comprises 7% to 10% of pancreatic cancer.
DCR, disease control rate; ORR, overall response rate; PR, partial response; SD, stable disease.

CHAPTER 6

Rare Gastrointestinal Tumors

Van Karlyle Morris and Ben George

Anal

With approximately 9000 cases are expected to occur annually (1), squamous cell carcinoma of the anal canal is considered a rare malignancy, but nonetheless is one which continues to rise in incidence (2). Most cases are linked to prior infection with high-risk human papilloma virus (HPV)—most commonly, HPV-16 and HPV-18. Historically, systemic cytotoxic therapy has been utilized in the management of patients with advanced anal cancer. In recent years, molecular characterizations of this tumor type have elucidated possible targets for therapeutic intervention. This section details genomic and immune biomarkers of interest in the clinical management of patients with anal cancer.

Genomic Biomarkers

Whole-exome sequencing performed on a cohort of patients with metastatic anal cancer revealed activating mutations in the *PIK3CA* oncogene to be the most common alteration, present in 29% of cases (3). Amplifications in *PIK3CA* were seen in 88% of tumors. Commercially available gene sequencing panels that investigated across all stages of anal cancer have corroborated that *PIK3CA* is mutated in approximately 30% of all anal cancers (4,5). Interestingly, these findings are consistent with TCGA data that included other HPV-positive cancers including head/neck (6) and the cervix (7), both of which have *PIK3CA* mutations at similar frequencies. To date, no phosphoinositide 3-kinase (PI3K) inhibitors or mechanistic target of rapamycin (mTOR) inhibitors have been formally tested, specifically in patients with advanced anal cancer.

Unlike adenocarcinomas arising in the adjacent colon/rectum, anal cancers are characterized by rare mutations in the *KRAS*, *NRAS*, and *BRAF* oncogenes (3). Multiple series have reported that mutations in these genes occur in <5% of all anal cancers (4,5). Oncologists should recognize differences in biologic drivers and molecular profiling that distinguish colorectal cancer from nearby anal cancer when considering application of targeted therapies in the management of advanced cancers of the distal gastrointestinal tract. Given this predisposition for *KRAS/NRAS/BRAF* wild-type status for anal cancer, retrospective series have reported both safety/tolerability and antitumor activity of anti–epidermal growth factor receptor (EGFR) antibodies (mostly in combination with cytotoxic chemotherapy) (8), providing rationale for possible activity of this targeted therapy.

Immune Biomarkers

Anal cancers are also characterized by low tumor mutation burden (TMB), with multiple series estimating mean TMB below 10 mutations per megabase (Mb) of DNA sequenced (3,9). TMB-high status occurs in <10% of reported anal cancers (9). Although the U.S. Food and Drug Administration (FDA) has approved pembrolizumab in patients with advanced solid tumors featuring a TMB >10 mutations/Mb (10), prospective studies thus far have not validated TMB as a predictive biomarker for benefit with immunotherapy in patients with advanced anal cancer.

Anti–programmed cell death 1 (PD-1) antibodies have demonstrated modest efficacy in patients with metastatic anal cancer with responses in single-arm phase II clinical trials reading between 10% and 24% (11,12). Post hoc analyses have suggested increased benefit in patients whose tumors feature high expression of programmed death ligand 1 (PD-L1) and higher CD8[+] T-cell infiltration in pretreatment tumor specimens (11). However, responses have also been observed in PD-L1-negative anal cancer patients by immunohistochemistry (12). At this time, PD-L1 has not been demonstrated to be a validated predictive biomarker for benefit with immunotherapy in patients with metastatic anal cancer.

Actionable Target	Abnormality	Prevalence (%)	Clinical Experience with Targeted Agent
PD-1, PD-L1	Expression	61	Nivolumab (anti-PD-1 antibody) (11) • Phase II: Overall response rate 24%, median PFS 4.1 months Pembrolizumab (anti-PD-1 antibody) (12) • Phase II: Overall response rate 11%, median PFS 2.0 months Retifanlimab (anti-PD-1 antibody) (13) • Phase II: Overall response rate 14%, median PFS 2.3 months Avelumab (anti-PD-L1 antibody) (14) • Single agent: Phase II: Overall response rate 10%, median PFS 2.1 months • With cetuximab (anti-EGFR antibody): Overall response rate 17%, median PFS 3.9 months

EGFR, epidermal growth factor receptor; PD-1, programmed cell death 1; PD-L1, programmed death-ligand 1; PFS, progression-free survival.

Adenocarcinomas represent 25% to 40% of the 11,390 new cases of small bowel cancer reported annually in the United States (1,15,16). The incidence of adenocarcinoma is highest in the duodenum and decreases progressively throughout the rest of the small intestine (17,18). Systemic chemotherapy is the current mainstay of treatment for advanced small bowel adenocarcinomas (SBAs), but identification of predictive biomarkers to drive therapeutic decision-making is garnering increasing attention.

Mismatch repair deficiency (dMMR) status ranging from 1% to 16% has been reported for SBAs (19–21), although 7% to 10% of SBAs have high levels of TMB—defined as ≥20 mutations per megabase (21,22). A large series that prospectively analyzed samples from 317 patients with SBA identified *TP53, KRAS, APC, SMAD4, PIK3CA, CDKN2A,* and *ARID1A* as the most altered genes (>10% of cases), whereas *ERBB2* alterations (mostly point mutations) and *BRAF* mutations (mostly non-V600E) were identified in 9.5% and 9.1% of cases, respectively (21). Another study identified a 22% incidence of DNA damage repair (DDR) gene alterations (*ARID1A, ATM, ATR, BRCA1, BRCA2, CDK12, CHEK1, CHEK2, PALB2,* and *RAD51*) in 666 patients with SBAs (22). Further, exome sequencing performed on 106 primary SBAs demonstrated four mutational signatures—signature 6, associated with mismatch repair (MMR) deficiency; signature 1A, associated with older age; and signatures 17 and U2, with no specific associations (23). The genomic profile of SBAs, even while harboring some similarities to those of colorectal cancer and gastric cancer, appears to be driven by disparate and distinct driver alterations meriting individualized treatment approaches (21,23).

The phase II KEYNOTE-158 study demonstrated the efficacy of pembrolizumab in dMMR SBAs—among the 19 patients with SBA, there were eight objective responses (42%), three of which were complete, and the duration of response ranged from 4.3 to 13.3+ months (24). Pembrolizumab also has a tissue-agnostic FDA approval for the treatment of TMB-high (≥10 mutations/Mb) tumors, but the study that led to this approval did not enroll any patients with SBA (10). A prospective, multicenter, phase II study that investigated the role of pembrolizumab in SBAs demonstrated objective responses in dMMR (2/4; 50%) and TMB-high (≥10 mutations/Mb—2/2; 100%) patients but did not confer any benefit in unselected patients (25). PD-L1 expression status did not correlate with response in an exploratory analysis performed as part of this study (25). In addition, FDA has granted targeted tissue-agnostic approvals of checkpoint inhibitors for dMMR (19,26) and TMB-high tumors (10).

The data on efficacy of anti–epidermal growth factor receptor (EGFR) therapy in SBAs are limited and conflicting, with some suggestion of response either as a single agent or in combination with chemotherapy (27,28).

The widespread use of comprehensive genomic profiling, identification of several actionable genomic targets, and enrollment in tissue-agnostic, biomarker-driven clinical trials will accelerate the prospective validation of personalized therapies for SBAs.

Appendiceal Cancer

Epithelial neoplasms of the appendix include invasive adenocarcinomas (AAs) and goblet cell adenocarcinomas (GCAs). They are rare with an incidence of <1 per 100,000 population (29). In the absence of prospectively validated data, systemic chemotherapy for patients with appendiceal adenocarcinomas largely follows treatment for metastatic colorectal cancer.

One of the earliest and most comprehensive efforts at tissue-based molecular characterization of AAs tested tumor samples from 149 patients and demonstrated a molecular profile distinct from that of colorectal cancer (30). COX-2 expression, *KRAS*, *PI3K*, and *BRAF* mutations were seen in 61%, 55%, 17%, and 4% of patients, respectively, whereas microsatellite instability high (MSI-H) status was noted in 6% of patients (30). Therapy targeted against COX-2 and EGFR provided no clinical benefit in this series. Another comprehensive genomic profiling attempt using 588 samples of appendiceal tumors (77% AAs, 9% GCAs) identified mutations in *KRAS* (50.4%), *TP53* (21.9%), *GNAS* (17.6%), *SMAD4* (16.5%), *APC* (10%), *ATM* (7.5%), *PIK3CA* (5.5%), *FBXW7* (5.0%), and *BRAF* (1.8%) (31). A subsequent attempt at characterizing circulating tumor DNA (ctDNA)-based alterations in AAs correlated with alterations previously reported in tissue-based testing, suggesting the feasibility of noninvasive testing in these patients (32).

Neurotrophic tyrosine receptor kinase (NTRK) fusions are detected rarely (<1%) in appendiceal cancers meriting treatment with TRK inhibitors—larotrectinib and entrectinib (33,34). Currently, there are no other FDA-approved targeted therapies for AAs other than tissue-agnostic approvals of checkpoint inhibitors for dMMR (19,26) and TMB-high tumors (10).

Molecular alterations in uncommon GI cancers and therapy

Histology	Actionable Target	Prevalence (%)	Therapy
Small bowel adenocarcinoma	dMMR	1–16	Pembrolizumab (12,35) Phase II: ORR 34.3% (12), 39.6% (35) PFS 4.1 months Dostarlimab (36) Phase 1: ORR 38.7% PFS NA
	TMB high (≥10 mutations/mega base)	8–12	Pembrolizumab (10,37) Tissue agnostic approval (based on response rate and durability of response) Approval was based on data from the KEYNOTE-158 trial. Across all tumor types, ORR 29%, CR 4%. The median DOR was not reached, with 57% of pts having response durations ≥12 months and 50% of pts having response durations ≥24 months.
	NTRK fusion	–	Larotrectinib (34,38) Tissue agnostic approval (based on response rate and durability of response) Approval was based on data from three multicenter, open-label, single-arm clinical trials: LOXO-TRK-14001, SCOUT, and NAVIGATE; across all tumor types, ORR 75%, CR rate 22%.

(continued)

Histology	Actionable Target	Prevalence (%)	Therapy
			At the time of database lock, median DOR was not reached. Response duration was 6 months or longer for 73%, 9 months or longer for 63%, and 12 months or longer for 39% of pts. Entrectinib (39,40) Tissue agnostic approval (based on response rate and durability of response) Approval was based on data from three multicenter, single-arm, clinical trials: ALKA, STARTRK-1, and STARTRK-2; across all tumor types, ORR 57%, DOR was 6 months or longer for 68% of pts and 12 months or longer for 45% of pts.
Appendiceal cancer	dMMR	6	Pembrolizumab (12,35) Tissue agnostic approval (based on response rate and durability of response) Approval was based on data from 149 pts with MSI-H or dMMR cancers enrolled across five uncontrolled, multicohort, multicenter, single-arm clinical trials. Across all tumor types, ORR 39.6%, CR 7%.

Histology	Actionable Target	Prevalence (%)	Therapy
			Responses lasted 6 months or more for 78% of those who responded to pembrolizumab. Dostarlimab (36) Tissue agnostic approval (based on response rate and durability of response) Approval was based on GARNET Trial, a nonrandomized, multicenter, open-label, multicohort trial. Across all tumor types, ORR 38.7%, CR 9.1%. Median DOR was 34.7 months with 95.4% of pts with duration ≥6 months.
	TMB high (≥10 mutations/mega base)	2–3	Pembrolizumab (10,37) Tissue agnostic approval (based on response rate and durability of response) Approval was based on data from the KEYNOTE-158 trial. Across all tumor types, ORR 29%, CR 4%. The median DOR was not reached, with 57% of pts having response durations ≥12 months and 50% of pts having response durations ≥24 months.

(*continued*)

Histology	Actionable Target	Prevalence (%)	Therapy
	NTRK fusion	<1	Larotrectinib (34,38) Tissue agnostic approval (based on response rate and durability of response) Approval was based on data from three multicenter, open-label, single-arm clinical trials: LOXO-TRK-14001, SCOUT, and NAVIGATE; across all tumor types, ORR 75%, CR rate 22%. At the time of database lock, median DOR was not reached. Response duration was 6 months or longer for 73%, 9 months or longer for 63%, and 12 months or longer for 39% of pts.
			Entrectinib (39,40) Tissue agnostic approval (based on response rate and durability of response) Approval was based on data from three multicenter, single-arm, clinical trials: ALKA, STARTRK-1, and STARTRK-2; across all tumor types, ORR 57%. DOR was 6 months or longer for 68% of pts and 12 months or longer for 45% of pts.

CR, complete response; dMMR, deficient mismatch repair; DOR, duration of response; MSI-H, microsatellite instability high; NA, not available; NTRK, neurotrophic tyrosine receptor kinase; ORR, overall response rate; PFS, progression-free survival; TMB, tumor mutation burden.

Malignant Peritoneal Mesothelioma

Malignant peritoneal mesothelioma (MPM) is a rare disease—only 10% to 15% of the mesotheliomas diagnosed in the United States are peritoneal, accounting for approximately 600 cases per year (41,42). There are different histologic subtypes—the sarcomatoid or biphasic subtype has a worse prognosis than the more common epithelial subtype (43,44). Because of the rarity of this entity, lack of robust, prospectively validated clinical trials, and heterogeneous clinical behavior of MPM, there is no consensus on the optimal systemic therapy for this disease.

A subset of patients with MPM may harbor germline or somatic alterations in the mismatch repair (MMR) genes, suggesting putative response to immunotherapy (45–48). Identification of anaplastic lymphoma kinase (ALK) rearrangements in MPM (3%) along with a few reports of response to molecularly targeted therapy in this subgroup merits prospective evaluation (49–53).

The role of immunotherapy in MPM is evolving. MPM harbors a complex immune milieu and a proinflammatory microenvironment with PD-L1 expression reported in approximately 50% to 60% of cases (54,55). Prospective studies that evaluated checkpoint inhibition either as a single agent or in combination with chemotherapy have not yet reported convincing activity in the MPM subset (56–58). However, a recent phase II trial of 20 patients with advanced MPM and progression or intolerance to prior platinum-pemetrexed chemotherapy demonstrated encouraging activity to a combination of atezolizumab and bevacizumab (59). The confirmed objective response rate (primary endpoint) was 40%, median duration of response was 12.8 months, and responses were independent of PD-L1 overexpression, or presence of dMMR status (59).

Currently, there are no FDA-approved targeted therapies for MPMs other than tissue-agnostic approvals for dMMR (22,30) and TMB-high tumors (10).

Histology	Actionable Target	Prevalence	Therapy
Malignant peritoneal mesothelioma	dMMR	<5%	Pembrolizumab (12,35) Tissue agnostic approval (based on response rate and durability of response) Approval was based on data from 149 pts with MSI-H or dMMR cancers enrolled across five uncontrolled, multicohort, multicenter, single-arm clinical trials. Across all tumor types, ORR 39.6%, CR 7%. Responses lasted 6 months or more for 78% of those who responded to pembrolizumab. Dostarlimab (36) Tissue agnostic approval (based on response rate and durability of response) Approval was based on GARNET Trial, a nonrandomized, multicenter, open-label, multicohort trial. Across all tumor types, ORR 38.7%, CR– 9.1%. Median DOR was 34.7 months with 95.4% of pts with duration ≥6 months.

Histology	Actionable Target	Prevalence	Therapy
	TMB high (≥10 mutations/ mega base)	–	Pembrolizumab (10,37) Tissue agnostic approval (based on response rate and durability of response) Approval was based on data from the KEYNOTE-158 trial. Across all tumor types, ORR 29%, CR 4%. The median DOR was not reached, with 57% of pts having response durations ≥12 months and 50% of pts having response durations ≥24 months.
	NTRK fusion	–	Larotrectinib (34,38) Tissue agnostic approval (based on response rate and durability of response) Approval was based on data from three multicenter, open-label, single-arm clinical trials: LOXO-TRK-14001, SCOUT, and NAVIGATE; across all tumor types, ORR 75%, CR 22%. At the time of database lock, median DOR was not reached. Response duration was 6 months or longer for 73%, 9 months or longer for 63%, and 12 months or longer for 39% of pts.

(continued)

Histology	Actionable Target	Prevalence	Therapy
			Entrectinib (39,40) Tissue agnostic approval (based on response rate and durability of response) Approval was based on data from three multicenter, single-arm, clinical trials: ALKA, STARTRK-1, and STARTRK-2; across all tumor types, ORR 57%. Response duration was 6 months or longer for 68% of pts and 12 months or longer for 45% of pts.

CR, complete response; dMMR, deficient mismatch repair; DOR, duration of response; MSI-H, microsatellite instability high; NTRK, neurotrophic tyrosine receptor kinase; ORR, overall response rate; TMB, tumor mutation burden.

CHAPTER 7

Cancer of Unknown Primary

Nicholas James Hornstein, Ryan Huey, and Kanwal Pratap Sing Raghav

Introduction

- Cancer of unknown primary (CUP) represents a heterogeneous group of metastatic cancers wherein the primary site of origin eludes detection despite adequate and recommended diagnostic workup (1–3).
- Although CUP is a well-recognized clinical entity characterized by an unusual pattern of metastatic spread distinct from other cancers with known primaries, the central oncogenic mechanisms that underlie this "atypical cancer syndrome" are unclear to date.
- Consequently, the controversy regarding the validity of CUP diagnosis persists: irresolutely between CUP being an erroneous diagnosis because of inadequate diagnostics to detect a primary lesion and being a distinct biologic entity sharing molecular features (4,5).
- Although early transcriptomics showed CUP to be discrete from metastases of known origin, the range of genomic aberrations appears to be similar and shared between both entities (6,7).
- These conflicting views are reflected in the differing management paradigms for this disease, expressly separated into two camps: "site-specific therapy" wherein treatment is modeled after the most likely putative primary and "empiric chemotherapy" with combined broad-spectrum cytotoxic chemotherapy, notably carboplatin and paclitaxel (Figure 7.1).
- Regardless of genesis, patients with CUP present a challenge in oncology clinics because of the heterogeneity of presentation, complexity of diagnostic workup, and few treatment options.
- Although the era of molecularly targeted therapies and immunotherapies has seen significant advances in systemic therapy for cancers with known primary, progress in CUP has lagged because of limited CUP-specific research and exclusion from tumor-specific clinical trials.
- In this chapter, we will review the current management of CUP and the promise of novel targeted and immune therapies in the treatment of this poorly understood and orphan disease.

Epidemiology and Prognosis

- Because of advances in imaging, pathology, and molecular profiling, the incidence of CUP has declined over the past few decades (8). Cancers traditionally misdiagnosed as CUP, such as cholangiocarcinoma, germ cell tumor, and certain sarcomas, are increasingly distinguished from CUP with improved immunohistochemistry, cytopathology, and molecular diagnostics.

Figure 7.1   71

Proposed algorithm for the management of cancer of unknown primary (CUP). Patients with CUP should have detailed clinical, radiographic, and pathologic workup. All patients eligible for treatment should have molecular profiling performed. Treatment can be either site-specific where the workup indicates a putative primary or empiric cytotoxic chemotherapy or molecularly directed therapy. Participation in clinical trials should be always encouraged.

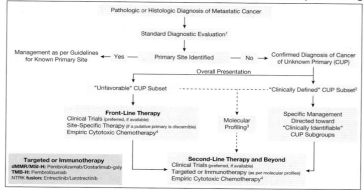

[1] Standard diagnostic evaluation includes comprehensive clinical examination (history, physical and blood [± tumor markers]), optimal radiologic workup (CT chest, abdomen, and pelvis with intravenous contrast, unless contraindicated [± focused use of MRI or PET-CT]), and adequate pathologic evaluation (morphology and immunohistochemistry). Tissue-of-origin profiling is not standard but maybe used in select cases or in clinical trials.

[2] "Clinically defined" CUP subsets have been historically known as "Favorable" CUP subsets and include women with primary peritoneal carcinomatosis (s/o serous carcinoma) or adenocarcinoma with axillary lymph node involvement, men with bone metastases and elevated prostate-specific antigen (PSA), extragonadal germ cell tumors, and neuroendocrine carcinoma.

[3] Molecular profile (tissue or blood) should ideally include next-generation sequencing (NGS) and markers for FDA-approved tissue-agnostic approvals (immunotherapy for tumors with deficient mismatch-repair [dMMR] or high microsatellite instability [MSI-H] or high tumor mutation burden [TMB-H] and TRK inhibitors for tumors harboring NTRK gene fusions).

[4] Commonly used empiric cytotoxic chemotherapy includes regimens such as carboplatin + paclitaxel, gemcitabine + cisplatin/carboplatin.

- CUP is a rare cancer with an incidence of 4 to 6 cases per 100,000 population in the United States and constitutes roughly 2% of all cancer diagnosis (8,9). An estimated 32,880 new cases of CUP will be diagnosed in the United States annually (10). This grouping of "CUP patients" is a mix of tumors with diverse histologies and varying biology and clinical behavior.
- CUP is classified into broad histologic categories based on light microscopy; adenocarcinoma of unknown primary (ACUP) is most frequent, representing about 70% to 75% of CUP cases, whereas squamous cell carcinoma of unknown primary (SqCUP) and undifferentiated carcinoma constitute approximately 6% to 9% and 25% to 35% of all CUP cases, respectively (8,11,12).
- With limited therapeutic options, the overall prognosis of patients with CUP has remained poor (8). Globally, the median survival of all patients with CUP ranges from 2 to 3 months (8,11,12).
- Survival is strongly dependent on histology, with 1-year survival rates of 15% to 17% for ACUP to 53% for SqCUP (8). Corresponding 5-year survival rates are 6% and 41%, respectively (8). Sarcomatoid CUP (SCUP) is another aggressive histology with poor overall survival (13).
- Additionally, other factors like gender, Eastern Cooperative Oncology Group (ECOG) performance status (PS), histology, number of metastatic sites (and sites of metastatic spread), and neutrophil–lymphocyte ratio also impact prognosis (8,11,12,14). Clinical subsets such as lymph node–only disease (LNCUP) have a better overall survival (median: 33 months) compared to those with bone-predominant (BCUP) disease (median 15 months) or patients with other CUP (median: 16 months) (15).

Molecular Profiling and Tissue (Site) of Origin

- Historically, CUP was regarded as a distinct form of cancer, related more biologically than anatomically, and treated as such with empiric therapy (16–20). Over the years, there has been a shift in this belief toward the notion that CUP may be a metastatic cancer syndrome wherein the metastatic tumors may retain the essence of their original tissue of origin (ToO) (21,22).
- Pathologic evaluation, especially tumor-specific immunohistochemistry, is commonly used for labeling CUP, vis-à-vis tumor lineage and identifying a primary site, though this strategy is not helpful in all patients because of limits of sensitivity and specificity of various markers (23–25).

- Advances in molecular profiling (gene expression and microRNA profiling) led to the development of several platforms designed to identify the ToO, on the premise that a cancer classifier built using discriminatory markers from cancers of known primaries can predict ToO in CUP (26).
- Common ToO assays used clinically have been based on either gene expression or microRNA profiling (27–30). These classifiers were initially developed and validated on samples derived from both primary and metastatic tumors of known primary cancers. The challenge of direct validation in CUP remains because of the absence of a gold standard diagnostic.
- Assay performances in CUP were determined by level of agreement with putative primary profiles based on clinicopathologic features and latent primary and therapy response (31–33). ToO assays agreed with putative primary calls in 61% to 94% of successfully processed samples (31–34).
- With next-generation sequencing (NGS) permeating the management of cancers with known primary, expanded efforts in CUP using genomics and transcriptomics coupled with machine learning algorithms have been used to develop novel ToO prediction assays with increased ability to predict ToO in 50% to 97% of patients with CUP (35–38).
- The decisive objective of accurate identification of a ToO is to aid in optimizing patient management based on the assumption that a "site-specific therapy" will improve outcomes of CUP patients compared to a shotgun approach of "empiric therapy."
- Two prospective outcome-based studies have examined the role of ToO assays to direct site-specific therapy in patients with CUP; one was a randomized trial.
- In the first study, a 92-gene assay successfully predicted ToO in 85% of CUP cases and most commonly identified biliary tract (18%), urothelium (11%), and colorectal (10%) sites (39). The median survival of patients who received assay-directed site-specific treatment was 13 months and correlated with the therapeutic responsiveness of assay-predicted tumor types (39).
- However, the randomized trial evaluating ToO assay (using gene expression profiling)–directed site-specific therapy vs. empiric chemotherapy (carboplatin–paclitaxel) failed to show any significant improvement in 1 year (44% vs. 55%) (40).
- Key guidelines do not endorse routine clinical use of ToO assays in the management of CUP because of unproven impact of assay-defined primary site-specific therapy on patient outcomes (2,3).

Empiric Treatment in CUP

- An alternative to site-specific treatment in CUP is empiric therapy. Although multiple regimens have been investigated, it is unclear if any regimen is superior compared to others.
- A meta-analysis of 32 relevant studies on chemotherapeutics in unfavorable CUP showed a trend toward better survival outcomes with platinum- or taxane-based regimens (41). Median and 1-year survival rates seen were 9 to 10 months and 37% to 41%, respectively. Hence, use of carboplatin and paclitaxel as empiric therapy in CUP is widely recommended (40).

Molecular Profiling and Targeted/Immune Therapy

- The idea of molecular or genomic-directed therapy improving outcomes in pan-cancer tissue-agnostic settings, for instance, targeting *ERBB2* (*HER2*) amplification, irrespective of tumor type (e.g., breast, gastric, colon, and biliary tract) is driven by some successes, and has pervaded the cancer treatment paradigm and inspired similar efforts in CUP (42).
- In large studies of NGS data from CUP samples (both tissue and blood), 80% to 95% of patients harbored at least one genomic alteration (Figure 7.2) (7,43,44). These alterations were different between ACUP and non-ACUP (7). Among these, 15% to 99% of alterations have been considered potentially targetable or druggable, which highlights the heterogeneity of population and subjective definitions of "actionability" (7,44–47).
- The molecular profile of CUP is minimally stereotyped, with significant heterogeneity amid patients. *TP53* mutations are most common (42%) followed by *KRAS* (19%) (Figure 7.2) (46). Alterations where a U.S. Food and Drug Administration (FDA)-approved therapy for a cancer of known primary exists occur in a small subset of CUP patients, such as *HER2* amplifications (3%–4%); *BRAF* (2%–4%), *EGFR* (5%–6%), and *IDH1* mutations (2%–5%); and *FGFR2* fusions (1%) (7,44).
- Furthermore, predictive biomarkers of response to immunotherapy have been seen in about 28% of all CUP patients, with programmed death ligand 1 (PD-L1) expression seen in 22% of cases (43).
- Alterations with tissue-agnostic FDA approval such as deficient-mismatch repair (dMMR) or microsatellite high (MSI-H) status or high tumor mutation burden (TMB-H) are seen in 12% and 2% of CUP cases, whereas NTRK gene fusions are seen in <1% patients (Table 7.1) (43,48).

Figure 7.2

75

Common genomic alterations seen in cancer of unknown primary (CUP). Patients with CUP can present with a plethora of genetic alterations. The relative significance with regard to their oncogenic or "driver" potential and thereby the value of targeting these genetic alterations is unclear in CUP. The figure represents the prevalence of various alterations as reported in three large series of patients with CUP who underwent comprehensive sequencing.

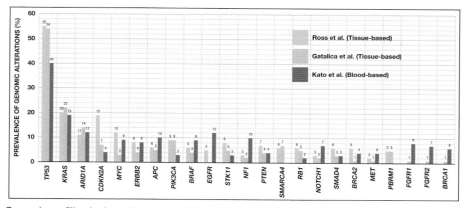

Genomic profiling in these three large series of CUP patients using tissue-based or blood-based clinical laboratory improvement amendments (CLIA)-certified assays (7,3,44). Genomic alterations (mutations and copy number variations) occurring in = 5% of patients/samples and in at least two of these three series were included for illustrating the prevalence.

- Efforts utilizing genomic sequencing to guide treatments in CUP have demonstrated encouraging clinical benefit with sequencing-directed therapy (30%–50%) in some case series, highlighting the promise of targeted therapies (35,45,46,49).
  - The CUPISCO randomized phase II trial (NCT03498521) is expected to provide a prospective comparison of molecularly guided therapy vs. platinum-based chemotherapy in patients with newly diagnosed "unfavorable" CUP (50).
- Early evidence from phase II trials has demonstrated an objective response rate of approximately 23% with single-agent immune checkpoint agents (pembrolizumab or nivolumab) in an unselected CUP patient population (51,52). However, data are limited in CUP, and these regimens lack FDA approval or indication for use.
- The feasibility of NGS in CUP is frequently limited because of inadequacy and quality of tissue, as samples often undergo extensive testing as part of diagnostic workup. Insufficient tissue was cited as the reason for screen failure in CUPISCO in 25.7% of patients and is higher in real-world populations (50,53). Blood-based (circulating tumor DNA) assays can help overcome this handicap (44).

Approved Targeted/Immune Therapies for CUP

- No specific targeted or immune therapy is approved for CUP barring recent pan-cancer FDA approvals for tissue-agnostic drug approvals for all advanced solid tumors (Table 7.1).
- Pembrolizumab was approved for dMMR/MSI-H or TMB-H, and tropomyosin receptor kinase (TRK) inhibitors (larotrectinib and entrectinib) were approved for NTRK gene fusion harboring advanced solid tumors that have progressed following prior treatment and have no satisfactory alternative treatment options. Details of these approvals are provided in Table 7.1. Notably, only few CUP patients were treated in trials that led to approval of these agents (2,3,54–56).
- We believe that despite the limited data today, the future of CUP treatment will be shaped by its underlying genomic and immunologic milieu. Although off-label use of both targeted and immune therapy has been promoted in some patients with CUP because of limited treatment options, this is not available or useful to a large section of this populace.
- We believe that integrating molecular profiling in initial workup to identify potential actionable targets and early referral of CUP patients to clinical trials are much needed to better understand this rare and capricious entity, and to truly advance the standard of care for CUP patients toward improved outcomes in this orphan disease.

	Cancer of Unknown Primary (CUP)		
Actionable Target	Abnormality	Prevalence (%)	Clinical Experience with Targeted or Immunotherapy Agent
PD-1	Deficient-Mismatch Repair (dMMR) or Microsatellite High (MSI-H)	1.8 (43)	**Dostarlimab-gxly (PD-1 inhibitor):** • FDA approved (2021) for all patients with MSI-H or dMMR advanced solid tumors • Phase I GARNET study (NCT02715284) *(N = 106) (57)*: ORR: 38.7% (95% CI: 29.4, 48.6), 18-month DOR: 80.9%, CUP patients: *N = 1* (PR) **Pembrolizumab (PD-1 inhibitor):** • FDA approved (2017) for all patients with MSI-H or dMMR advanced solid tumors • Five uncontrolled, multicohort, multicenter, single-arm clinical trials *(N = 149) (58)*: ORR: 39.6% (95% CI: 31.7, 47.9), 6-month DOR: 78%, CUP patients: *N = NS* • Phase II KEYNOTE-158 study (NCT02628067) *(N = 233) (59)*: ORR: 34.3% (95% CI: 28.3, 40.8), 24-month DOR: 77.6%, CUP patients: *N = NS*
PD-1	High Tumor Mutational Burden (TMB-H)	11.8 (43)	**Pembrolizumab (PD-1 inhibitor):** • FDA approved (2020) for all patients with TMB-H advanced solid tumors (TMB ≥ 10 mut/mb) • Phase II KEYNOTE-158 study (NCT02628067) *(N = 102) (54)*: ORR: 29% (95% CI: 31, 39), 24-month DOR: 67%, CUP patients: *N = NS*

(continued)

Cancer of Unknown Primary (CUP)

Actionable Target	Abnormality	Prevalence (%)	Clinical Experience with Targeted or Immunotherapy Agent
NTRK	NTRK gene fusion	0.41 (48)	**Entrectinib (TRK/ROS/ALK inhibitor):** • FDA approved (2019) for all patients with advanced solid tumors with NTRK gene fusion • Three multicenter, single-arm, clinical trials (ALKA, STARTRK-1 [NCT02097810], and STARTRK-2 [NCT02568267]) (*N* = 54) (55): ORR: 57% (95% CI: 43.2, 70.8), 12-month DOR: 45%, CUP patients: *N* = NS **Larotrectinib (TRK inhibitor):** • FDA approved (2018) for all patients with advanced solid tumors with NTRK gene fusion • Three multicenter, single-arm, clinical trials (LOXO-TRK-14001 [NCT02122913], SCOUT [NCT02637687], and NAVIGATE [NCT02576431]) (*N* = 55) (56): ORR: 75% (95% CI: 61, 85), 12-month DOR: 71%, CUP patients: *N* = NS

DOR, duration of response; FDA, U.S. Food and Drug Administration; N, number of patients; NS, not specified; NTRK, neurotrophic tyrosine receptor kinase; ORR, overall response rate; PD-1, programmed cell death protein 1; PR, partial response; 95% CI, 95% confidence interval.

CHAPTER 8

Neuroendocrine Cancer

Daniel M. Halperin and Thorvardur R. Halfdanarson

In this chapter, we will consider the relevant targets and therapies for gastrointestinal neuroendocrine cancers. Although these malignancies are complex and nuanced, our hope would be to simplify the topic and associated medical decision-making.

Classification

Within the gastrointestinal tract, neuroendocrine neoplasms (NENs) are a heterogeneous family of malignancies with distinct manifestations and clinical outcomes, dependent on the site of origin, stage of disease, and pathologic grading (1). Pathologic grading uses a system elaborated in 2019 by the World Health Organization (2), which separates NENs into well-differentiated neuroendocrine tumors (NETs) and poorly differentiated neuroendocrine carcinomas (NECs). Well-differentiated NETs are further separated into grades 1 to 3 based on their replicative rate, as assessed by Ki-67 staining or mitotic index, whereas poorly differentiated NECs are universally grade 3.

The history of targeted therapies in NENs is paradoxically rife with success and failure. On the one hand, there are no genomic alterations that predict outcome with any approved standard therapy, making the utility of molecular profiling in standard practice rather modest. However, with the exception of alkylating chemotherapy for NETs arising in the pancreas (3,4), all available therapies in NETs are specific to molecular targets. In contrast, NECs lack actionable targets and are treated exclusively with cytotoxic chemotherapy as the standard of care.

Targeted Therapies

Well-differentiated NETs can boast one of the oldest and best-validated targets by virtue of their somatostatin receptor (SSTR) expression. For decades, radiolabeled somatostatin analogues have been incorporated into diagnostic techniques for tumor localization (5), and receptor expression has been considered a biomarker for response (6). Although receptor expression was mandatory for inclusion in the more modern CLARINET trial of lanreotide in patients with gastroenteropancreatic NETs (GEP-NETs) (7), it was not required in the PROMID study of octreotide for midgut patients, though the majority of patients did have known SSTR expression (8). Therefore, SSTR expression as assessed with modern nuclear imaging (e.g., DOTATATE PET) is considered as supportive of, but not required for, therapy with conventional somatostatin analogues, such as lanreotide or octreotide. In contrast, confirmation of receptor expression is required prior to peptide receptor radionuclide therapy (PRRT) such as ^{177}Lu-DOTATATE.

Although SSTR expression remains a putative predictive biomarker for conventional and radioactive somatostatin analogues, other targeted agents lack known predictors of response. Multiple inhibitors of vascular endothelial growth factor (VEGF) have been evaluated, though few of these agents have been studied in randomized trials. In pancreatic NETs, sunitinib was evaluated in a randomized study after a phase II trial using objective response rate as its primary endpoint only demonstrated volumetric reduction in NETs originating in the pancreas. Similarly, surufatinib, which has a somewhat broader spectrum of kinase inhibition, demonstrated significant reduction in the risk of progression or death when compared to best supportive care in patients with advanced, progressive panNET (SANET-p) (9). However, in a parallel study in patients with progressive extrapancreatic NETs (SANET-ep), surufatinib demonstrated similar efficacy (10), suggesting a disconnect between rates of tumor shrinkage and improvements in survival. The results of the SANET trials may not apply to the NET population in the United States given differences in the study populations, but relatively few patients with small bowel NETs were included and the patients were relatively lightly pretreated. Similarly, a randomized phase II study of pazopanib in patients with progressive extrapancreatic NET suggested improved progression-free survival compared to best supportive case, despite a 0% response rate in a single-arm phase II trial (11). Despite these clear benefits with VEGF-targeted tyrosine kinase inhibitors (TKIs), mutations in the genes of the VEGF pathway are rarely identified in NET, especially those arising outside the pancreas.

Similarly, the mechanistic target of rapamycin (mTOR) inhibitor everolimus was evaluated in a series of studies in patients with pancreatic and extrapancreatic NETs. In pancreatic tumors (12) and nonfunctional extrapancreatic tumors (13), everolimus demonstrated significant reduction in the risk of progression or death estimated to be 65% and 52%, respectively. Another randomized clinical trial of everolimus in patients with extrapancreatic NET and carcinoid syndrome suggested improved progression-free survival (PFS) in patients treated with everolimus as compared to placebo but failed to meet its prespecified endpoint of efficacy (14). However, mutations in the mTOR pathway are rare (particularly in extrapancreatic NETs [15]) and have not been associated with benefit to our knowledge.

Immunotherapy

Finally, it is worthwhile to comment on the use of immunotherapy in both well-differentiated NET and poorly differentiated NECs of the gastrointestinal tract. Studies of single-agent checkpoint inhibitors in well-differentiated NET patients have been largely disappointing, with response rates and PFS durations similar to those observed with placebo (16–18). Results have been similarly challenging for patients with poorly differentiated NEC (18,19), although there has been some enthusiasm based on the results of the dual anti-CTLA-4 and anti-PD-1 blockade in rare tumors (DART SWOG 1609) study (20), which suggested that the combination of ipilimumab and nivolumab could induce responses in 8 of the 18 patients with G3 NENs of any primary site treated in the study. Results from larger studies of this combination in more homogeneous patient populations are eagerly anticipated to potentially impact standard of care.

Conclusion

Although poorly differentiated NECs remain poorly targeted with modern therapies, well-differentiated NET patients have seen substantial benefit from treatments directed at their specific phenotypic features, even if no new predictive biomarkers have been identified since somatostatin receptors were identified three decades ago. With continued characterization, it remains hopeful that we will see benefits from novel targeted and immunotherapies in the years to come.

Actionable Target	Abnormality	Prevalence (%)	Clinical Experience with Targeted Agent
SSTR2	Expression	~80 (potentially higher in some subgroups, e.g., midgut)	**Octreotide** (SSA binding SSTR2/5): • Phase III monotherapy with PFS HR 0.35 vs. BSC in treatment-naïve patients with midgut NET (8) **Lanreotide** (SSA binding SSTR2/5): • Phase III monotherapy with PFS HR 0.47 vs. BSC in treatment-naïve patients with GEP-NET (7) [177]**Lu-DOTATATE** (therapeutic radionuclide conjugated to SSA binding SSTR2/5): • Phase III monotherapy with PFS HR 0.21 vs. octreotide 60 mg in patients with midgut NET progressing on octreotide 30 mg (21)
VEGF			Sunitinib • Phase III monotherapy with PFS HR 0.42 vs. BSC in patients with progressive pancreatic NET (22) Surufatinib • Phase III monotherapy with PFS HR 0.49 vs. BSC in patients with progressive pancreatic NET (9) • Phase III monotherapy with PFS HR 0.33 vs. BSC in patients with progressive extrapancreatic NET (10)

(continued)

Actionable Target	Abnormality	Prevalence (%)	Clinical Experience with Targeted Agent
			Pazopanib • Randomized phase II monotherapy (87% concurrent SSA) with PFS HR 0.53 vs. BSC in patients with progressive extrapancreatic NET (23) Axitinib • Randomized phase I/II monotherapy (concurrent SSA in all) with PFS HR 0.71 vs. BSC in progressive extrapancreatic NETs (24)
mTOR			Everolimus • Phase III monotherapy with PFS HR 0.35 vs. BSC in patients with progressive pancreatic NET (12) • Phase III monotherapy with PFS HR 0.48 vs. BSC in patients with progressive extrapancreatic NET (13)

BSC, best supportive care; GEP-NET, gastroenteropancreatic neuroendocrine tumor; HR, hazard ratio; mTOR, mechanistic target of rapamycin; NET, neuroendocrine tumor; PFS, progression-free survival; SSA, somatostatin analog; SSTR, somatostatin receptor; VEGF, vascular endothelial growth factor.

Sequencing Technologies

CHAPTER 9
Introduction of High-Throughput Sequencing

Timothy Philip DiPeri and Funda Meric-Bernstam

Introduction

At the turn of the millennium, one of the largest breakthroughs in contemporary medical science was announced—the majority of the human genome had been sequenced, unveiling a new road map for human biology (1). Over the past two decades, sequencing technologies have advanced at a rapid pace, which has had broad implications for the detection and treatment of human disease (2). The field of oncology has been at the forefront of these developments, considering the relevance of genetics in cancer. High-throughput sequencing, or next-generation sequencing (NGS), has made comprehensive molecular profiling of cancers feasible and has profoundly changed our understanding of human tumor biology (3).

Although NGS was once considered cost-prohibitive and utilized sparingly for research efforts, it is now commonplace in oncology practices (4). This has given rise to the era of precision oncology, which refers to a personalized approach to cancer medicine by using an individual tumor's molecular characteristics to guide therapeutic decision-making (5). Rapid identification of alterations in cancer-related genes, which may have diagnostic, prognostic, and/or therapeutic relevance, has revolutionized modern cancer care. In this chapter, we will introduce high-throughput sequencing by reviewing the historical context into the sequencing of the cancer genome, discussing platforms to detect alterations within the genome and transcriptome, how high-throughput sequencing data can be leveraged for the treatment of cancer patients, and challenges with integrating these data into clinical practice.

Sequencing the Cancer Genome

Shortly after completion of the Human Genome Project, several international efforts were launched to comprehensively profile a diverse set of cancers and to gain insight into tumorigenesis, most notably The Cancer Genome Atlas (TCGA) and International Cancer Genome Consortium (ICGC) (6,7). Although many oncogenic drivers/tumor suppressors had previously been identified, it was clear that an understanding of the spectrum of genomic aberrations that drive cancers was imperative. The vision for the TCGA project, as put forth by the National Institutes of Health (NIH), was ambitious—multiple centers and a vast array of multiomics approaches were utilized to molecularly profile >30 different tumor types (8). Methods to acquire these data included RNA sequencing

(RNASeq), micro RNA sequencing (miRNASeq), DNA sequencing (DNASeq), single-nucleotide polymorphism (SNP)-based platforms, and array-based DNA methylation sequencing for nucleic acid sequencing, as well as reverse-phase protein array (RPPA) for proteomic assessment (6). Subsequently, the TCGA Pan-Cancer project was implemented and sought to further analyze the molecular profiles of individual tumors, as well as compare genetic aberrations between tumor types (8). Similarly, the ICGC characterized >50 cancer types, with the goal of discovering highly prevalent mutations, standardizing reporting methods on an international scale, providing granular data at the single-nucleotide level, and to make this data publicly accessible (7).

Progress in the field of cancer biology that has stemmed from these efforts cannot be overstated. The field of oncology was previously predominated by a tumor-centric approach to treatment, but it is now evident that tumors with vastly different origins can have overlapping molecular drivers, and often tumors of the same origin are molecularly distinct (8). Publicly available data from the TCGA and ICGC have allowed researchers around the globe to make progress in identifying biomarkers, discovering new targets for therapy, and providing an opportunity to develop bioinformatics tools to better understand the available data, which will ultimately improve the care of cancer patients (6).

Detection of Genomic Alterations

High-throughput DNASeq can be performed using several molecular biology techniques, including cyclic reversible termination, pyrosequencing, synthesis by ligation, and real-time sequencing (9). Sequences determined by these assays are then mapped onto the human reference genome using bioinformatics tools, which enables the calling of single-nucleotide variants, insertions/deletions, fusions, and copy number variations (Figure 9.1). These NGS technologies are advantageous over first-generation Sanger sequencing, considering that the volume of data that can be produced with one run can exceed 1 billion short reads (9). Tissue input for these assays includes solid tumor tissue, individual tumor cells, and plasma (liquid biopsy). Although fresh frozen tissue provides adequate tissue for performing NGS, samples are often formalin fixed and paraffin embedded (FFPE), which can lead to the degradation of both DNA and RNA (10). Despite these limitations, most modern NGS platforms can utilize FFPE tissue for sequencing analysis.

Figure 9.1

89

Flowchart of genomic and transcriptomic assessment using NGS. DNA, deoxyribonucleic acid; Mb, megabase; NGS, next-generation sequencing; RNA, ribonucleic acid.

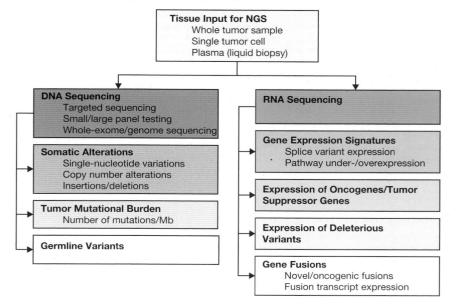

Several NGS platforms have emerged, which may be encountered by oncologists, including commercially available/adapted platforms, institutionally developed platforms, and research-based platforms. Sequencing platforms vary widely and may refer to targeted and small panels of <100 genes, large panels of >100 genes, whole-exome sequencing (WES)/whole-genome sequencing (WGS), and RNASeq. Many commercial platforms have emerged for tumor or tumor-normal sequencing, including FoundationOne CDx, Caris CDx, TempusXT, and Oncomine Comprehensive Assay (11). Some institutions have also adapted these assays for in-house profiling efforts, whereas others have developed their own sequencing platforms, such as the Memorial Sloan Kettering-Integrated Mutation Profiling of Actionable Cancer Targets (MSK-IMPACT) platform, which is a hybridization capture–based assay (12). WES and WGS are still less frequently performed but provide additional data that are not confined to genes covered on a single panel and are often used in a research-based setting.

With the increasing prevalence of large panel testing in oncology, a question that is often encountered in practice is whether or not an alteration is germline (present in all or most tissue) or somatic (present in tumor cells but not in other tissues). Importantly, panels are not able to distinguish if a variant is germline or somatically acquired, if tumor-only testing was performed, rather than tumor paired with a matched normal sample (such as blood). Additionally, when germline variants are identified, there is a lack of consensus on which genes may warrant germline-focused analysis and, furthermore, what degree of penetrance is required to determine cancer risk. Groups such as the European Society of Medical Oncology (ESMO) Precision Medicine Working Group (PMWG) have established guidelines for germline-focused analysis to allow oncologists to navigate these challenging clinical questions (13).

Unveiling the Transcriptome

Transcriptomics is broadly defined as the analysis of messenger RNA (mRNA), ribosomal RNA (rRNA), transfer RNA (tRNA), micro RNA (miRNAs), and long non-coding RNAs (ncRNAs). High-throughput transcriptional sequencing by RNASeq gives precise details on base pair sequences and additional RNAs that cannot be identified with the conventional microarray technology (14). Following the isolation of RNA from a given tissue, it is then converted to complementary DNA (cDNA) by reverse transcription and further amplified by polymerase chain reaction (PCR) to allow for the detection of RNA sequences (15). The clinical utility of transcriptional profiling is evolving and is a component of tumor biology that should be taken into consideration in parallel with genomic profiling efforts. RNASeq is advantageous as it can allow for the detection of unique isoforms/splice variants, gene expression signatures, and fusions/rearrangements (14). Differential gene expression in cancer pathways can have downstream effects that potentiate tumor growth, often without corresponding genomic alterations, which may highlight avenues for therapeutic intervention (16). In addition to gene expression signatures, RNASeq also can identify gene fusions and fusion transcript expression, which have prognostic, and diagnostic, implications and have been emerging as some of the most compelling therapeutic targets in precision oncology (16).

Personalized Cancer Therapy

Progress in the field of genomic medicine has profoundly improved our understanding of cancer biology and ushered in the era of precision oncology. NGS is now routinely performed at both academic and community cancer centers and can inform oncologists of which molecular characteristics are driving a tumor that may have therapeutic relevance. Early successes in precision oncology are highlighted by the benefits of trastuzumab in HER2-positive breast cancer (17) and vemurafenib in BRAF V600E mutant melanoma (18), among others. A study from the MD Anderson Cancer Center identified that in a phase I setting, patients treated with molecularly matched therapies had an improved overall response rate (27%) in comparison to those who received non-matched therapies (5%) (19). The phase II MyPathway study investigated if U.S. Food and Drug Administration (FDA)-approved therapies had activity across 14 different tumor types, and identified meaningful responses in 23% of patients with metastatic solid tumors when matched with agents outside of their FDA-approved indications (20). These findings are promising for cancer therapeutics, though a remaining challenge is the lack of FDA-approved therapies for most alterations. Basket trials are a way to address this concern through a tumor-agnostic approach to enrollment, which can facilitate the evaluation of matched therapies in patients with less common alterations.

The surplus of data acquired from broad-based sequencing efforts poses a set of new challenges for oncologists—how can this information be best incorporated into clinical practice to improve outcomes for patients? A survey of physicians at a National Cancer Institute (NCI)-designated comprehensive cancer center identified that physicians have varying levels of confidence regarding the incorporation of genomic data into practice (21). Although many genes have been identified that have prognostic and/or therapeutic relevance, there is a knowledge gap in determining if a particular alteration is a "driver" or "passenger," and which alterations may be clinically "actionable," meaning that they may be targeted directly or indirectly with investigational or approved agents (22). Integration of NGS data requires not only the accurate detection of genomic alterations but also an understanding of the clinical implications associated with an alteration, and awareness of trials that the patient may be eligible for (22). Furthermore, access to both multiplex genomic profiling and molecularly targeted therapies varies widely by institution (23). A study by Meric-Bernstam et al. reported that few patients with actionable alterations were ultimately enrolled in genotype-matched trials (23). Efforts to address these concerns include decision support programs to assess if a variant is actionable and/or affects eligibility criteria for an ongoing clinical trial (24). Several publicly available precision oncology resources have also been established to help provide insight into the actionability of alterations, including the MD Anderson Personalized Cancer Therapy website (www.personalizedcancertherapy.org) (25), the Cornell Precision Medicine Knowledge Base (PMKB) website (https://pmkb.weill.cornell.edu/) (26), and the Memorial Sloan Kettering OncoKB website (https://www.oncokb.org/) (27). These findings highlight the need for institutional, programmatic efforts to implement decision support for precision oncology to facilitate the enrollment of patients with actionable alterations into clinical trials.

Conclusion

High-throughput sequencing has revolutionized modern cancer care and enabled oncologists to routinely profile tumors in clinical practice. Clinical integration of genomic and transcriptomic data obtained from NGS is evolving, and decision support programs can be utilized to assess the functionality of a given aberration, which may facilitate clinical trial enrollment.

CHAPTER 10

Liquid Biopsies in Gastrointestinal Cancers

Shalini Makawita and Arvind Dasari

Introduction

In this section we will discuss liquid biopsies, specifically pertaining to cell-free DNA (cfDNA) or circulating tumor DNA (ctDNA), and its applicability in the management of gastrointestinal (GI) cancer patients.

Liquid biopsies are simple, noninvasive tests in biologic fluids such as blood or urine that enable the measurement of clinically relevant biomarkers. There are many analytes within the circulatory system that can serve as markers of disease states, such as proteins, messenger mRNA, micro RNA (miRNA), and cell-free DNA (cfDNA). cfDNA had been first reported in 1948 by Mandel and Metais in human plasma and consists of fragments of genetic material found outside of the cell (1). In 1977, Leon et al. (2) had reported elevated levels of cfDNA in cancer patients when compared to healthy individuals. cfDNA that has been released from tumor cells is referred to as ctDNA and can vary in range from a minute portion (<1%) of an individual's total cfDNA to a relatively high abundance correlating with tumor burden. cfDNA or ctDNA can serve as a surrogate marker of disease in cancer patients, and three potential mechanisms for its release into circulation have been described: necrosis, apoptosis, and active secretion (Figure 10.1) (3).

Over the past decades, with significant advancements in methods for ctDNA detection, its applicability in the clinical care of cancer patients has been garnering significant interest and research. This includes its use as prognostic and/or predictive markers, in the detection of disease recurrence after definitive therapy, in the management of minimal residual disease (MRD), in monitoring response to therapy, and in identification of resistance mechanisms after exposure to targeted therapies (Figure 10.1). Through sampling of the blood for ctDNA at multiple time points during a patient's cancer treatment, liquid biopsies can aid in the longitudinal evaluation of a patient's cancer genome. In the sections below, we detail clinical applications of ctDNA within the context of common GI malignancies.

Figure 10.1

95

Mechanisms of circulating tumor DNA (ctDNA) release and its applications in the care of gastrointestinal cancer patients. MRD, minimal residual disease.

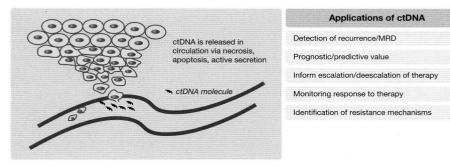

Colorectal Cancer

Several early studies by multiple groups had shown individual cfDNA markers or marker panels as well as methylation patterns to have the ability to distinguish patients with colorectal cancer (CRC) from benign or healthy controls. These early studies had also established good concordance with tissue molecular profiling (4,5). In a study where fresh frozen tissue and plasma samples obtained at the time of surgery from 29 CRC patients were analyzed with an 85-gene panel, median ctDNA levels of 14.2 and 8.94 ng/mL were noted in colon and rectal cancer patients, respectively, with 70% concordance between ctDNA and tissue molecular profile. The small number of rectal cancer patients in this study ($N = 10$) had lower overall concordance (50%) with tissue profiles (6). Systematic reviews of literature published over the past two decades have noted other individual ctDNA markers such as septin 9 (*SEPT9*), or marker panels, that have been studied for disease detection. Varying ranges of sensitivity (37%–96%) and specificity (79%–99%) among studies have excluded these markers as clinically useful screening tools but with potential for other applications such as disease monitoring with further validation (7). Methylation status of promoter regions of genes methylguanine methyltransferase (*MGMT*) and DNA excision repair protein (*ERCC-1*) analyzed via liquid biopsy in 50 patients with rectal cancer compared to 43 patients with benign rectal lesions had also shown discriminatory potential with a specificity of 93% to 95% and sensitivity of approximately 60% (8). Petit et al. (7) from their systematic review concluded that methylated cfDNA may serve as a promising candidate for CRC detection.

With the advent of next-generation sequencing (NGS), genomic profiling using various commercially available liquid biopsy platforms has enabled serial analysis of ctDNA for prediction of survival outcomes and detection of disease recurrence. MRD is defined as minute amounts of cancer cells remaining during or after completion of therapy as detected by highly sensitive techniques. MRD can imply the presence of micrometastasis prior to clinical detection. Identification of ctDNA after definitive surgery in colon cancer patients has been associated with increased disease recurrence. In a study of 231 stage II colon cancer patients, ctDNA had been detected in 14/178 patients postoperatively who did not receive adjuvant therapy, and 11/14 (79%) patients had recurrence of disease at 27 months follow-up compared to a recurrence rate of 16/164 (9.8%) patients who did not have ctDNA present postoperatively (hazard ratio [HR] 18; 95% confidence interval [CI] 7.9–40;

$p < 0.001$) (9). In patients who received adjuvant chemotherapy, ctDNA positivity directly after completion was associated with worse recurrence-free survival (RFS) (HR 11; 95% CI 1.8–68; $p = 0.001$). Reinert et al. (10) used ultradeep multiplex polymerase chain reaction (PCR)-based NGS sequencing of ctDNA in their prospective multicenter cohort study of 130 patients with stage I–III CRC at selected time points, including before surgery, on postoperative day 30, and once every 3 months for up to 3 years to evaluate its utility in detecting clinical recurrence and RFS. Using WES of tumor to identify 16 highly ranked somatic single-nucleotide variants and short indels, this group used a technology to construct personalized liquid biopsies for each patient. Preoperatively, 88.5% of patients had detectable ctDNA. Post-op ctDNA positivity was associated with seven times more likelihood of relapse (HR 7.2; 95% CI 2.7–19.0; $p < 0.001$), and ctDNA positivity after adjuvant chemotherapy was associated with 17 times more likelihood of relapse (HR 17.5; 95% CI 5.4–56.5; $p < 0.001$). Currently, although such assays are predictive of survival outcomes, prospective clinical trials are needed to determine if intervention with additional therapy based on ctDNA detection will improve these outcomes.

Currently, the standard of care is to offer adjuvant chemotherapy after surgical resection for patients with stage III colon adenocarcinoma and high-risk stage II disease (T4, inadequate lymph node harvest [≤12], tumors complicated by obstruction or perforation, poorly differentiated or vascular/perineural or lymphatic invasion) (11). There are no validated biomarkers in standard clinical practice for identification of MRD after surgical resection in colon cancer; however, ongoing prospective studies incorporating ctDNA analyses are underway to inform clinical decision-making with regard to adjuvant therapy. In the prospective phase II/III COBRA trial (NCT04068103), patients with stage IIA disease without high-risk features after surgical resection who are deemed candidates for observation and no systemic chemotherapy will be randomized 1:1 to observation or prospective testing of ctDNA for both colon cancer–relevant genetic mutations and methylation profiling (12). Those in the ctDNA arm with detectable ctDNA will be treated for 6 months with adjuvant 5-fluorouracil, leucovorin, oxaliplatin (FOLFOX)/capecitabine, oxaliplatin (CAPOX) chemotherapy. Primary endpoints of this study include the clearance of ctDNA with use of adjuvant systemic therapy and RFS in patients with detected ctDNA treated with or without systemic therapy.

Other clinical trials exploring the utility of ctDNA for informing adjuvant chemotherapy include the Australian DYNAMIC III study (ACTRN12617001566325) in stage III colon cancer, and the CIRCULATE-Japan and US trials (NCT04120701) (13). Data from the observational GALAXY study within CIRCULATE-Japan evaluating a total of 1,365 patients with stage I–IV CRC showed improved 6-month disease-free survival (DFS) rate in patients with positive ctDNA at 4 weeks who turned negative at 12 weeks post-op ($N = 58$) compared to those whose ctDNA remained positive at 4 and 12 weeks ($N = 78$) (DFS 100% vs. 45%; HR 52.3; $p < 0.001$). Clearance of ctDNA at 12 weeks was significantly higher in those who received adjuvant chemotherapy (57% vs. 8%, all stages $p < 0.001$), and 6-month DFS rate was significantly higher in ctDNA-positive patients who received adjuvant chemotherapy (84% vs. 34%; HR 0.15; $p < 0.001$) (14,15). ctDNA informed therapy escalation/deescalation is ongoing. These studies are summarized in Table 10.1.

ctDNA (MRD positivity) has also shown to be prognostic in patients with oligometastatic colon cancer. In a cohort of 112 patients with metastatic CRC (mCRC) from the PREDATOR clinical trial, ctDNA was positive in 54.4% of patients postoperatively (median testing at 27 days post-op; range 8–99.5 days) (16). Approximately 97% of patients with MRD had progressed at time of data cutoff (HR 5.8; 95% CI 3.9–68; $p < 0.001$). MRD-positive patients also had lower overall survival. MRD-positive patients that had not received postoperative chemotherapy had a markedly reduced DFS (HR 15; 95% CI 4.3–49; $p < 0.001$). MiRDA-C (minimal residual disease assessment in patients with CRC, NCT04739072) is an ongoing prospective observational clinical trial evaluating ctDNA levels at baseline, during neoadjuvant therapy, prior to surgery, and during surveillance to determine feasibility and ability of MRD/ctDNA to improve detection of recurrence after completion of curative-intent therapy. Similar to colon cancer, the presence of ctDNA detected in locally advanced rectal cancer (LARC) patients postoperatively is a strong indicator of recurrence of disease. In a study of 47 patients with localized rectal cancer who underwent chemo-radiotherapy (CRT) followed by resection with serial plasma sampling, ctDNA was detected in 74% pretreatment, 21% mid- and post-CRT, and 13% postoperatively (17). Post-CRT ctDNA levels were associated with magnetic resonance imaging (MRI) tumor regression, and metastasis-free survival was shorter in those with detectable ctDNA post-CRT (HR 7.1; 95% CI 2.4–21.5; $p < 0.001$) compared to those with undetectable ctDNA. In another study of LARC, detection of ctDNA postoperatively was a strong

Table 10.1: Selected prospective randomized clinical trials of ctDNA to inform clinical decision-making

Clinical Trial	Description	Primary Endpoints and Results
COBRA (NCT04068103) Phase II/III colon cancer	• Stage IIA colon cancer without high-risk features[a] 1:1 to SOC observation (Arm A) or prospective testing for ctDNA (Arm B). • Arm B: if detectable ctDNA post-op, then 6 months adjuvant chemotherapy	• ctDNA clearance with adjuvant therapy • RFS for Arm B **Results:** Study ongoing
DYNAMIC II (ACTRN12615000381583)	• Stage II CRC randomized 1:1 for treatment based on ctDNA result (Arm A) vs. SOC per physician (Arm B). • Arm A: if detectable ctDNA post-op, then 5-fluorouracil-based chemo	• Does ctDNA-based adjuvant therapy decision affect number of patients who receive chemotherapy, and RFS? **Results:** Study ongoing
DYNAMIC III (ACTRN12617001566325) Phase II/III colon cancer (Australia)	• Stage III colon cancer randomized 1:1 per post-op ctDNA (Arm B) or SOC (Arm A). Stratified for low (T1-3N1) and high (T4 or N2) risk. • Arm B: ctDNA negative managed with deescalation adjuvant treatment and ctDNA positive with escalation adjuvant strategy.	• Evaluate impact of deescalation/escalation ctDNA-based strategies. **Results:** Study ongoing

(continued)

Table 10.1: Selected prospective randomized clinical trials of ctDNA to inform clinical decision-making (*continued*)

Clinical Trial	Description	Primary Endpoints and Results
CIRCULATE-US (NRG-GI008)	• Stage II/III MSI-S CRC postresection. If ctDNA is negative, SOC adjuvant chemo vs. observation with serial ctDNA. If ctDNA is subsequently detected, or positive post-op, randomized to SOC chemo or intensified mFOLFOXIRI.	• DFS of ctDNA negative (immediate vs. delayed chemo) and ctDNA positive (SOC vs. intensified chemo) **Results:** Study ongoing

CIRCULATE-JAPAN	• Three clinical trials:
	  ○ GALAXY: prospective observational trial—stage II–IV CRC amenable for curative surgery
	  ○ VEGA: randomized phase III—test noninferiority of surgery alone to SOC CAPOX in HR stage II/LR stage III in ctDNA negative CRC
	  ○ ALTAIR: double-blind, phase III—trifluridine/tipiracil vs. placebo in ctDNA-positive CRC after completion of adjuvant chemotherapy
		• GALAXY: ctDNA dynamics, 6-month DFS rate
		• Results for GALAXY:
		  ○ Improved 6-month DFS 100% vs. 45% (HR 52.3; $p < 0.001$) if ctDNA+ 4 weeks post-op and negative at 12 weeks, compared to remaining positive at 12 weeks.
		  ○ 6-month DFS improved if ctDNA + and with adjuvant chemo (84%) vs. no chemo (34%, $p < 0.001$)
		• VEGA: DFS
		
		Results: Study ongoing
		
		• *ALTAIR: DFS*
		
		Results: Study ongoing

Abbreviations: CRC, colorectal cancer; ctDNA, circulating tumor DNA; DFS, disease-free survival; HR, high risk; LR, low risk; MSI-S, microsatellite stable; RFS, recurrence-free survival; SOC, standard of care.
[a]High-risk features: T4 disease, inadequate lymph node harvest (≤12), tumors complicated by obstruction or perforation, poorly differentiated, or vascular/perineural or lymphatic invasion.

predictor of disease recurrence despite adjuvant chemotherapy (18). In such patients, though there is a prognostic implication, there is currently no defined clinical role for the use of ctDNA to inform further cancer-directed therapy after completion of total neoadjuvant or adjuvant therapy, warranting its incorporation into future neoadjuvant and adjuvant therapy trials for clinical validation.

Longitudinal monitoring of relative variant allele frequencies of specific genes is also being used to inform therapy. For instance, acquired *RAS* and *EGFR* mutations monitored serially in patients after progression on anti-epidermal growth factor receptor (EGFR) therapies have shown exponential decay in these mutations, which can lead to rechallenge strategies of anti-EGFR therapies (19).

Pancreatic Cancer

In pancreatic cancer, ctDNA has been shown to have diagnostic potential in differentiating pancreatic ductal adenocarcinoma (PDAC) from other pancreatic neoplasms and benign pancreatic conditions such as chronic pancreatitis (20,21). In a prospective study designed to evaluate the diagnostic accuracy of cfDNA in pancreaticobiliary patients using NGS of a 54-gene panel in both tumor and plasma-derived cfDNA, 13 of 26 (50%) patients were found to have 100% concordance between tissue and cfDNA, with an additional 12% showing partial concordance. Overall, 90.3% of mutations detected in tissue samples were also detected in cfDNA. Diagnostic accuracy of cfDNA was noted to be 97.7% with 92.3% sensitivity and 100% specificity for a panel of five genes (22). Subsequent studies have also demonstrated detection of ctDNA at diagnosis and postoperatively to be an indicator for worse overall survival. In patients who had undergone curative pancreatoduodenectomy, detection of *KRAS* mutations in ctDNA was associated with significantly worse median overall survival compared to those without detectable ctDNA (13.6 vs. 27.6 months, respectively). Multiple other studies have shown detection of postoperative ctDNA to be correlated with shorter DFS (21). In a study of 93 patients with resectable, borderline resectable, and unresectable disease each having a median of three ctDNA assessments, ctDNA positivity occurred at a rate of 49.5%. RFS correlated strongly with postoperative ctDNA positivity (HR 8.0; $p = 1.6e-6$) (23). Adjuvant therapy trials with use of ctDNA to potentially escalate or deescalate therapy based on risk stratification are clinically warranted. Other applications for ctDNA in pancreatic cancer include monitoring response to therapy and surveillance of disease with the potential for early detection of recurrences. In addition to ctDNA analytes for liquid biopsies, circulating tumor cells and extracellular vesicles and exosomes detectable in the circulation are also being studied in pancreatic cancer with similar clinical applications (21,24).

Gastric Cancer

Similar to the other cancer types, increased levels of cfDNA have been significantly associated with gastric cancer compared to benign or healthy controls in multiple studies. Levels were found to correlate with advanced stage and tumor size >5 cm. cfDNA has also been shown to be more sensitive at disease detection in comparison to conventional markers such as carcinoembryonic antigen and CA19.9 (25). In a large-scale analysis of 1,005 patients with stage I–III disease of eight common cancer types, including gastric and esophageal, a combination of eight known protein markers with use of a 61-amplicon panel querying 16 genes that included *TP53*, *KRAS*, *PIK3CA*, *APC* (CancerSEEK panel) was used to study early detection when compared to 812 healthy controls. With application of rigorous statistical analyses, this panel had shown median 70% sensitivity at specificity of >99% for detection of all eight cancer types; however, sensitivity for this assay had been limited to 40% for early-stage disease partly limited by the abundance of analytes in circulation in early-stage disease (26). Methylation patterns of ctDNA-detected genes have also been evaluated and hypermethylation of several genes including RunX3, RPRM, and RASSF1A has been associated with early-stage gastric cancer, though no clinically validated tests currently are in routine use (27). Copy number variants of cMYC and HER2 have also been detected via ctDNA analysis. Though its utility in gastric cancer detection is limited by its overall low prevalence in this patient population, a recent study demonstrated its utility in monitoring response to therapy in HER2-amplified gastric cancer and identifying new alterations that emerged with development of resistance to therapy, which can help to inform subsequent line therapies for these patients (28). Incorporation of ctDNA into prospective clinical trials in this setting is warranted with standardization of ctDNA amplification criteria and interpretation.

Hepatobiliary

In biliary tract cancers (BTCs), approximately 40% to 50% of patients have targetable alterations, and treatment has become more precision oncology driven. Although the sensitivity and concordance between liquid and tissue biopsy have improved in this patient population, now up to 80% to 90% with two samples in driver genes, assay characteristics are still limited for it to serve as a diagnostic tool (29). In patients in whom sufficient cytologic or tissue sampling is not possible for molecular profiling, ctDNA-detected targetable alterations can inform therapy. In BTC, liquid biopsies can also serve as a means for disease monitoring on targeted therapy and detecting acquired resistance mutations through serial measurements in patients who have baseline ctDNA positivity (29). Serial liquid biopsies in three patients who were treated with infigratinib, the small molecule FGFR inhibitor, in the phase II clinical trial had shown multiple point mutations in the kinase domain of FGFR2 in postprogression analysis (30). Such serial monitoring can aid in tailoring subsequent therapy to overcome resistance (31).

In hepatocellular carcinoma (HCC), cfDNA with alfa-fetoprotein (AFP) in 24 patients with HCC and 62 patients with chronic hepatitis B with varying levels of fibrosis was able to distinguish HCC with a sensitivity and specificity of 87% and 100%, respectively, using what the authors referred to as HCC index (cfDNA, AFP, and age) (32). cfDNA from patients with HCC is more fragmented and shorter than in those with benign liver conditions and patients without liver disease. Methylation patterns, single-nucleotide mutations, and chromosomal rearrangements have been associated with disease detection. The CancerSEEK panel described earlier had shown 98% sensitivity and 99% specificity for distinguishing 44 HCC patients from 812 healthy controls (26). These panels require additional rigorous validation studies with incorporation of benign diseases before they would be ready for clinical practice (33).

Challenges to Liquid Biopsies

We have outlined the potential uses of ctDNA in various GI malignancies. In most cancer types, studies have shown the ability to distinguish disease from controls with varying sensitivity and specificity. Challenges to bringing these tools to the clinic include the limit of detection of assays coupled with low levels of ctDNA related to tumor burden, particularly for the early detection of disease. Approximately 6,000 diploid genomic molecules are present in 4 mL of plasma, providing a sensitivity limit of 0.01%. Improvements in assay sensitivity with ultradeep sequencing techniques and use of NGS panels that enable use of large numbers of epigenetic and genetic markers are facilitating improvements in sensitivity. Preanalytical considerations for ctDNA analysis have been described previously (34).

Other practical considerations of selecting and developing liquid biopsy platforms with high sensitivities (>95%) in order to detect very low tumor burden in the context of surveillance or MRD with maintaining high specificity (>99%) would be important to avoid false negatives and undertreatment of patients. On the other hand, DNA aberrations from hematopoietic stem cells released into circulation increase with increasing age and can give rise to alterations in genes such as *KRAS* and *TP53*, which are also found in CRC and thereby can contribute to false positives. The concomitant use of bioinformatics tools to parse ctDNA-based genomic profiling can assist in limiting these incidences. Controlling for lead-time bias in these studies would be an important factor as well. These and other important practical considerations are discussed in greater detail in the recent whitepaper set forth by the National Cancer Institute colon and rectal-anal task forces (13).

CHAPTER 11

Immune Landscape of Gastrointestinal Malignancy

Maggie Phillips and Gregory B. Lesinski

Introduction

Gastrointestinal (GI) tumors harbor a series of distinct immunologic features and are comprised of heterogeneous immune cell populations. The origins of many GI malignancies are closely related to inflammatory pathology, which may influence the landscape of cytokines, chemokines, and cellular constituents of these tumors. The failure of both endogenous and immunotherapy-induced antitumor immune responses across a range of GI malignancies is multifactorial. Several factors intrinsic to T cells themselves, such as inhibitory immune checkpoint receptors, or extrinsic to the T cells, including cytokines, chemokines, or suppressive cell types, comprise a redundant network that limits antitumor immunity. This dominant, suppressive immune phenotype can be characterized by canonical skewing of cytokine and chemokine profiles, paired with limited effector T-cell infiltration and a predominance of myeloid-lineage cells. Finally, the complexity of the microenvironment within GI tumors is also reflected in heterogeneous cancer-associated fibroblast (CAF) populations that facilitate cross-talk with both tumor and immune cells to regulate disease progression. This chapter provides an overview of key immunologic features of GI malignancies and provides a perspective related to priorities for future multidisciplinary research to advance the field.

The Microenvironment of GI Tumors Harbors Cellular Complexity

Malignancy can develop across multiple organ sites within the GI system, leading to aggressive tumors, many of which harbor key immunologic features. Complex cellular interactions with the immune system influence the course of disease and the response to immunotherapy (1). Thus, there is clinical importance in understanding the biology behind *why* these tumors are inherently nonresponsive to immunotherapy. Ultimately this could enable innovative treatment approaches for overcoming barriers to efficacy. One notable feature across GI cancer types is the striking cellular heterogeneity that exists within the tumor microenvironment (TME). It is now appreciated that a diverse array of cell populations can cooperate with transformed cells, further amplifying their aggressive behavior or shielding them from elimination by endogenous immune cells (Figure 11.1) (2). Key cellular components of the TME encompass vasculature, such as pericytes or endothelial cells,

Figure 11.1

107

The tumor microenvironment (TME) of gastrointestinal (GI) cancers. The TME comprises complex interactions between both cellular and soluble components. Cellular cross-talk between immune cells, cancer-associated fibroblasts, and cancer cells can dictate disease progression and therapeutic response. These cellular components additionally secrete soluble factors, like chemokines and cytokines, that further influence the inflammatory TME of GI cancers.

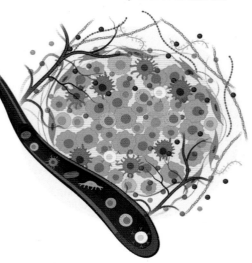

Cancer-Associated Fibroblast (CAF)

Dendritic Cell (DC)

Natural Killer (NK) Cell

Tumor-Associated Macrophage (TAM)

Myeloid-Derived Suppressor Cell (MDSC)

T Cell

B Cell

Cancer Cell

Pericyte

Extracellular Matrix (ECM) Proteins

Chemokines and Cytokines

the immune system, including lymphocytes or myeloid cells and fibroblast populations (3). Notably, CAFs play a major role in facilitating cross-talk and remodeling the architecture of the tumor and its surrounding stroma (4). This chapter will provide a brief overview on key immunologic features of GI tumors and our current understanding as to the role of various cellular components and soluble factors in this setting.

Inflammation Shapes the Immunologic Profile of GI Tumors

Given their anatomic origins, a salient feature present among most GI tumors is a close link with inflammatory pathology. There are many examples illustrating this relationship, including connections with viral infections and hepatocellular carcinoma, liver fluke infections with cholangiocarcinoma, Crohn's- and colitis-associated colorectal cancer, and pancreatitis with pancreatic ductal adenocarcinoma (PDAC) (5–8). Furthermore, it is becoming increasingly appreciated that inflammation in the GI tract occurs concomitantly with alterations in the microbiome that may further impact cancer risk (9–13). Inflammation most certainly brings about dynamic change in GI tissues that are subject to oxidative damage, fibrosis, and an influx of lymphocytes, myeloid cells, and other innate immune cells that essentially render a failed attempt at restoring tissue homeostasis and repair (14). Together with underlying genomic aberrations in the epithelial cells residing in GI organs, this scenario perpetuates cellular transformation and tumor formation.

Cytokines and Chemokines Perpetuate the Inflammatory Nature of GI Tumors

The relationship between inflammation and GI malignancy clearly influences cytokine and immune cell profiles observed in these tumors. Dynamic interplay between cytokine or chemokine mediators is important for shaping the composition of immune cells within GI tumors. Many cytokines and chemokines are present at high levels either systemically in patients with GI tumors or within the TME. There is a high degree of redundancy in the functional consequences of this cytokine and chemokine dysregulation, which culminates in a suppressed antitumor immune response. Some cytokines of notable importance in the setting of GI tumors that are supported by data from the literature include transforming growth factor-β (TGF-β), interleukin-6 (IL-6), IL-8, and vascular endothelial growth factor (VEGF), among others (15–18). In general, cytokine profiles are skewed away from the Th1 type, which can promote optimal immune responses from cytotoxic T and natural killer (NK) cells. Instead, Th2 and Th17 signatures are far more common in these patients, which enable maintenance of functionally suppressive immune cells including T regulatory cells (T regs), myeloid-derived suppressor cells (MDSC) or M2-polarized, tumor-associated macrophages (TAMs) (19–21).

Other evidence supports a role for cytokines in the colony-stimulating factor family, such as granulocyte macrophage-colony-stimulating factor (GM-CSF), granulocyte-colony-stimulating factor (G-CSF), and macrophage-colony-stimulating factor (M-CSF), which enable preferential expansion of myeloid cells (22,23). Parallel to these immune changes, tumors confer other biologic advantages from cytokines and growth factors that enable angiogenesis including basic fibroblast growth factor (bFGF), IL-8, and VEGF. Using VEGF as an example, many of these factors can simultaneously influence multiple facets of the TME by concurrently enabling blood vessel formation and acting via its receptor that is expressed on immune cells to further promote expansion of T regs and MDSC. This cytokine profile can also be coupled with dysregulation of chemokine gradients in a manner that preferentially attracts suppressive immune cells. For example, GI tumors and their stroma can produce CXCL12/SDF-1 that limits access of T cells into the TME (24).

Data also continue to emerge linking distinct oncogenic driver mutations in tumor cells with production of specific chemokine mediators. One prominent example of this was from Li et al., who demonstrated oncogenic *KRAS* can enable myeloid infiltration in a manner that was dependent upon CXCL1 production by the tumor cells (25). Other connections between Wnt/β-catenin signaling or LKB1 mutations and reduced T-cell infiltration have also been noted (26,27). These observations support the idea that individualized immune signatures in the TME are subject to influence by the genomic features of the tumor itself.

Redundant Mechanisms of Immune Suppression Are Evident in GI Tumors

In general, many GI tumors are what is considered "immunologically cold," meaning they lack abundant effector T-cell infiltrates. This is likely due to multiple factors, including but not limited to poor availability of neoantigens in tumors, inadequate chemokine gradients to enable their trafficking, or T-cell apoptosis upon entry into the hostile TME (20). Often, effector T cells are sequestered in regions distant from tumor cells, and those T cells that do gain access display phenotypic properties consistent with exhaustion. Other data indicate T-cell subsets including T regs or Th17 cells are present in these tumors, and may contribute to the impaired antitumor immune response. In contrast, myeloid cells and macrophages are major components within GI malignancies (28–30). These cells may be derived from tissue resident populations or alternatively are home to the microenvironment via the circulation. Taken together, the cellular composition of GI tumors enables multiple redundant mechanisms that inhibit productive antitumor immune responses. In general terms, mechanisms of limiting antitumor T-cell-mediated immune responses can be subdivided into two categories: (1) mechanisms that are *intrinsic* to the T cell itself (i.e., T-cell intrinsic) or (2) those mediated *extrinsic* soluble or cellular factors in the environment that feed back to limit T-cell function (i.e., T-cell extrinsic).

T-Cell Intrinsic Mechanisms Can Limit Antitumor Immune Responses

The most notable T-cell intrinsic mechanisms of suppressed antitumor immune responses are exemplified by inhibitory immune checkpoint receptors present on the surface on immune cell populations including T cells. Indeed, a wealth of knowledge is now available regarding the mechanism by which targeting the inhibitory programmed cell death protein 1 (PD-1) receptor and its interactions with ligands programmed death ligand-1 (PD-L1) and PD-L2 can perpetuate exhaustion phenotypes in T cells upon chronic antigen stimulation, thereby influencing antitumor immune response (reviewed in Pauken et al. [31]). The mechanism of action of these therapies is likely far more complex as both PD-1 and its ligands are expressed on several different cell types (32). Likewise, other inhibitory immune checkpoints such as cytotoxic T-lymphocyte-associated protein-4 (CTLA-4) emerge more proximal to T-cell priming (33). Thus, the expression of PD-1, CTLA-4, and numerous other inhibitory receptors on T cells can enable functional impairment of antitumor immunity, and do so via distinct mechanisms (Figure 11.2). Importantly, multiple inhibitory immune checkpoint receptors have been characterized on the surface of T cells beyond PD-1, and these are often concurrently expressed, emphasizing their redundancy in function to sustain an immunologic advantage to tumors (34).

T-Cell Extrinsic Mechanisms Hinder Immunity against GI Malignancy

Complementing these hard-wired, T-cell-intrinsic suppressive mechanisms are a host of other cell types that limit antitumor immune responses via forces that are "extrinsic" to the T cells themselves. As discussed earlier, the landscape of immune cells populating GI tumors is dictated by cytokine and chemokine mediators. The net result is a limited number of both effector T cells, as well as cells with capacity to present tumor antigen and mount productive immune responses (20). One relevant example of this is recent evidence for IL-6-dependent apoptosis of type I dendritic cells (DC1) in pancreatic tumors (35). Importantly, this likely occurs early during the course of disease progression, even at the stage of PanIN lesions, further contributing to inadequate T-cell responses against these tumors. Myeloid cells including MDSC and TAM are prominent cellular components across the spectrum of GI tumors and suppress T-cell-mediated antitumor immune responses via several concurrent mechanisms. These include secretion of immune modulatory cytokines including TGF-β that directly limits cytotoxic capacity of T and NK cells, IL-10 that limits DC maturation and IL-6 that can promote MDSC expansion, and skewed T-cell profiles toward either T reg or Th17 phenotypes, depending on the other cytokines present (Figure 11.3) (36,37).

Figure 11.2

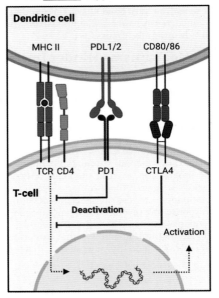

Figure 11.3

113

T-Cell <u>Extrinsic</u> Suppressive Mechanisms

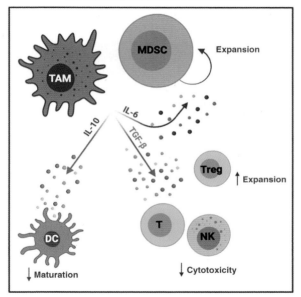

In a similar manner, B cells have been noted to secrete the cytokine IL-35 in several GI malignancies, resulting in exclusion of CD8$^+$ T cells from the tumor (38,39). In addition to cytokine mediators, suppressive immune cells can serve as potent regulators of metabolic features within the TME. There are many examples of this (reviewed in Lyssiotis et al. [40]) including lactate, indoleamine-pyrrole 2,3-dioxygenase-mediated tryptophan catabolism, production of arginase and cysteine deprivation, among others (41). More recently, attention has turned to immune cells with more innate properties including gamma delta T cells or innate lymphoid cells (ILC2) as additional components of the suppressive TME (42,43). The sheer redundancy in cellular and soluble factors likely emphasizes the need for combination therapy approaches to derive the best chance at success in aggressive GI malignancies (44).

CAFs: At the Crossroads of Communication between Tumor and Immune Cells

A deep appreciation for the role of CAFs in communicating with both the tumor and immune cells has more recently emerged. These cells reside across GI tumors of varied anatomic origin and a litany of publications have established their contributions to both fibrosis and immune suppression. However, it is important to note that many mechanistic assumptions related to CAF populations are derived from studies performed in pancreatic cancer. CAF populations have certainly been noted across other GI tumor types, including cholangiocarcinoma, colorectal cancer, hepatocellular carcinoma, and several others (45,46). The prevalence of these cells across disease settings emphasizes their importance in establishing and maintaining at least some common aspects of GI tumors, regardless of histology. Recent studies provide evidence for heterogeneity in inflammatory fibroblasts residing in tumor stroma (47–49). These data suggest that subpopulations of CAF can be defined based on alpha-smooth muscle actin (α-SMA) and IL-6, along with other markers. The topic of stromal components as promoting or inhibiting PDAC has definitely been a source of some controversy (50–52). For example, genetic ablation of SMA$^+$ stromal cells accelerated metastasis in a murine model of PDAC driven by oncogenic *Kras* (53). However, in this same tumor model, immunotherapy with anti-CTLA-4 antibody (Ab) was more effective when mice lacked SMA$^+$ cells

(53). Other animal studies have shown that fibroblast activation protein (FAP)-positive populations of CAF function to maintain stroma and suppress antitumor immune responses (24,54,55).

Aligned with the observations that cytokine profiles shape the immune cells present with tumors are data demonstrating another critical role for cytokines in regulating CAF plasticity. Using a series of organoid and other experimental models, Biffi et al. demonstrated that IL-1α and likely other factors from primary PDAC tumors promote an inflammatory CAF (iCAF) phenotype, whereas exposure of these same cells to TGF-β preferentially expands myofibroblast-like CAF (myCAFs) (56). iCAFs are defined via high IL-6 expression and are usually localized to fibrotic regions, more distant from adenocarcinoma in primary tumors. These iCAF cells promote immune suppression changes in the TME via IL-6 production (47,56). In contrast, myCAFs produce less IL-6 but express high levels of the α-SMA marker, and reside closer in proximity to malignant cells (47,56). Other heterogeneous CAF subsets have been assigned specialized functions, including the CD74+MHCII+ CAFs capable of presenting antigen to CD4+ T cells (57) or others expressing markers such as CD10 or CD105 (58,59). The advent of single-cell profiling technologies has also enabled discovery of other relevant targets on CAF (e.g., Col1A, NetrinG1, Lrrc15) and further subclassification of individual CAF subsets, along with more precise definition as to their origins (60–62). Finally, CAF-derived cytokines and chemokines are emerging as potential targets that can be leveraged to tune cross-talk with immune cells and augment response to immune therapy approaches. Several examples of this strategy are evident from the literature and include targeting IL-1, IL-6, CXCL12, placental growth factor, or TGF-β (24,63–66). Taken together, modulation of CAF, their soluble factors, and the key pathways governing their biologic properties hold promise for invigorating immune responses against GI malignancies.

Future Areas of Emphasis for Advancing Our Understanding of GI Tumor Immunology

There remains a pressing need to understand fundamental features that suppress antitumor immune responses in patients with GI malignancy. In concept, this would enable the field to prioritize novel, data-driven concepts that are common across different tumor types. Alternatively, this knowledge would allow for more precise discrimination of immune targets tailored to tumors with defined molecular or histologic features. Mirroring the experience with microsatellite unstable tumors and efficacy of PD-1/PD-L1 blockade antibodies in colorectal or other tumors, refining personalized approaches can impact care of patients (67). From a methodologic standpoint, more sophisticated spatially oriented and single-cell analyses are also undergoing continued refinement (68). Furthermore, continued deep sequencing approaches will enable better insight into the molecular features of tumors themselves (69). These tools will be powerful and enable rapid scientific advances.

Likewise, it will be imperative to continue efforts in developing better animal models, organoid technologies, and ensuring accessibility to human tissues in which to validate hypotheses in the clinical setting (70). Perhaps more consistent efforts at implementing clinical trials to test immunotherapy approaches in the neoadjuvant setting also hold value. Theoretically, this approach would ensure tissue access and direct investigation of therapeutic effects in the human setting. Further, it would enable intervention with immunotherapy approaches earlier during the course of disease and prior to multiple systemic exposures to chemotherapy. Another key limitation in the field is that much of our understanding into immune composition of GI tumors has been established from resection specimens, which capture carcinogenesis at an early to moderate stage. In contrast, across many tumor types, far less is known about the immune composition in the setting of metastasis. This may be particularly true for GI tumors that ultimately present with diffuse liver metastasis such as pancreatic cancer, whereby resection is not warranted and tissues for research and immunologic characterization are more limited. Finally, it is worth noting that great advances may arise from effective cross-disciplinary communication between scientists with diverse research interests and clinical investigators. The close links between cancer immunity with diet, obesity, the microbiome, and other emerging physiologic features are certainly worthy of deeper investigation. Unraveling these relationships in a mechanistic manner may hold important insight related to etiology, prevention, and therapy of GI cancer (71–73).

Molecular Targets and Pathways

An Introduction to the Organization of Cancer Cell Signaling

It is hard to do justice to the exquisite complexity of the cancer cell and to help comprehend the level of intra- and intercell signaling that occurs in the billions of cells in the human body. We have attempted to create an "org chart" to help classify the targets and strategies used to develop precision cancer treatment. There are three broad categories:

A. **Membrane Factors and Receptors (M 1–7):** Receptor Tyrosine Kinases (RTKs) for Survival Factors, Chemokines and Transmitters, and Growth Factors, the Extracellular Matrix, Fruit Fly Mutations, Death Receptors (DRs), and Cytokine Receptors

B. **Intracellular Systems (1–10):** Rapamycin, NF-Kappa B, G-Coupled Proteins, Mitogen-Activated Protein (MAP) Kinase (MAPK), SRC, β-Catenin, Caspases, Janus Kinase/Signal Transducer and Transcription (JAK/STAT), and Apoptosis

C. **Nuclear Factors, Cell Cycle Control, and DNA Repair (N):** MYC, Extracellular Signal–Regulated Kinase (ERK), Cyclins, Retinoblastoma (RB), MDM2, TP53

COLOR KEY

Agonist

Antagonist

Signal Transduction Roadmap

M1	Survival Factors/VEGF	C6	β-Catenin/APC
M2	Chemokines/Hormones	C7	Cell Regulators
M3	Growth Factors	C8	Caspases/BCL2
M4	Extracellular Matrix	C9	JAK/STAT
M5	Fruit Fly Receptors	C10	Apoptosis
M6	Death Receptors	N1	Extracell. Reg. Kinases
M7	Cytokines/Interleukins	N2	Cyclins
C1	Rapamycin/mTOR Sys	N3	Retinoblastoma/RB
C2	NF-Kappa B	N4	MYC
C3	G-Proteins/Cyclic AMP	N5	MDM2
C4	RAS→RAF→MAPKinase	N6	TP53/DNA Repair
C5	Sarcoma Gene—SRC	N7	Other Nuclear Factors

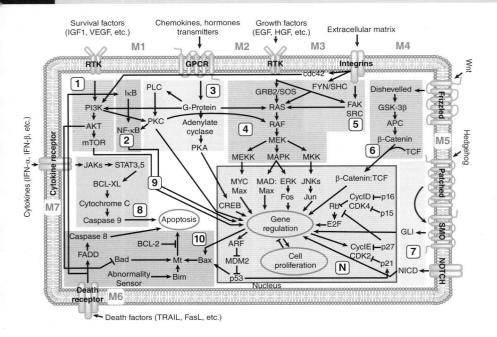

- Vascular endothelial growth factor (VEGF) is one of the most important and prominent proangiogenic factors. VEGF's normal function is to create new blood vessels during embryonic development, new blood vessels after injury, muscle following exercise, and new vessels (collateral circulation) to bypass blocked vessels.
- The VEGF family consists of five members (VEGF-A, -B, -C, -D, and placental growth factor [PlGF]), which transmit signals via three VEGF receptors (VEGFR-1 through VEGFR-3).
- Many human cancers are found to overexpress VEGFs and/or VEGFRs.
  - VEGFR-1 binding by VEGF-B plays a role in the maintenance of newly formed blood vessels.
  - VEGFR-2 activation by VEGF-A binding has been shown to stimulate endothelial cell (EC) mitogenesis and cell migration, leading to cancer progression and metastasis.
  - VEGFR-3 is predominantly expressed in lymphatic vessels. When bound by either VEGF-C or VEGF-D, VEGFR-3 plays a role in lymphangiogenesis and metastatic spread to lymph nodes in a pathologic setting.

Physiology	VEGF-A, -B, -C, -D and PlGF activate VEGFR-1, -2, -3 to promote vascularization
	• during embryogenesis • after injury
	• after vessel blockage • after exercise
Oncogenic VEGF, VEGFR behaviors	• Overexpressed in many cancers; expression associated with invasiveness, recurrence, prognosis
	• R2 activation by VEGF-A drives EC division and migration, and thus angiogenesis, cancer progression, metastasis.
	• R3 activation by VEGF-C, -D promotes metastasis to lymph nodes.

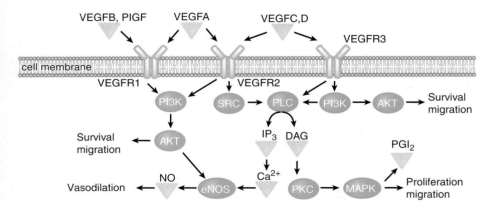

- Fibroblast growth factor receptor (FGFR) family has four highly conserved transmembrane RTKs (FGFR1–4) that differ in their ligand affinities and tissue distribution.
- Fibroblast growth factors (FGFs) include 18 structurally related polypeptides (FGF1–10, FGF16–23) that signal through FGFRs.
- FGFRs can bind canonical FGFs that are in complex with heparan sulfate proteoglycans (HSPGs) in an autocrine and paracrine fashion.
- FGFRs can also bind endocrine FGFs (FGF19, 21, and 23) that are found in circulation, free of HSPGs.
- Once bound to their ligands, FGFRs are induced to dimerize and cross-phosphorylate the tyrosine kinase domain on the cognate receptor.
- Various downstream effector molecules are then recruited, allowing for the activation of signaling events that culminate in regulation of various cellular processes such as cell survival and proliferation, organ development, angiogenesis, and tissue homeostasis, to name a few.
- Each FGFR can be activated by several FGFs; conversely, FGFs can activate more than one receptor.
- Dysregulation of FGFR signaling in cancer may be caused by the following:
  - *FGFR* gene amplifications, activating mutations, translocations, and fusions
  - Amplification of FGF and FGF-related genes
- Dysregulated FGFR signaling may contribute to cancer by the following:
  - Stimulating cancer cell proliferation
  - Driving tumor neovascularization
  - Promoting resistance to anticancer therapies

PHYSIOLOGY

- FGF1–10, FGF16–23 regulate essential cellular processes via FGFR1–4.
- Canonical FGFs elicit paracrine and autocrine effects.
- Others (FGF19, 21, 23) elicit endocrine effects.
- An FGF can trigger multiple FGFRs; an FGFR may engage several FGFs.
- Dysregulated signaling may promote cancer cell proliferation, tumor vascularization, and drug resistance.

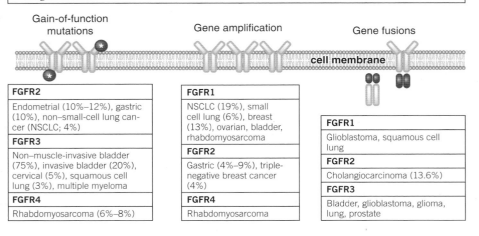

Gain-of-function mutations

FGFR2
Endometrial (10%–12%), gastric (10%), non–small-cell lung cancer (NSCLC; 4%)

FGFR3
Non–muscle-invasive bladder (75%), invasive bladder (20%), cervical (5%), squamous cell lung (3%), multiple myeloma

FGFR4
Rhabdomyosarcoma (6%–8%)

Gene amplification

FGFR1
NSCLC (19%), small cell lung (6%), breast (13%), ovarian, bladder, rhabdomyosarcoma

FGFR2
Gastric (4%–9%), triple-negative breast cancer (4%)

FGFR4
Rhabdomyosarcoma

Gene fusions

FGFR1
Glioblastoma, squamous cell lung

FGFR2
Cholangiocarcinoma (13.6%)

FGFR3
Bladder, glioblastoma, glioma, lung, prostate

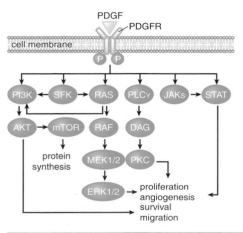

PHYSIOLOGY

- Platelet-derived growth factor (PDGF) A–D are potent mitogens for cells of mesenchymal origin.
- Synthesized, stored, and released by platelets upon activation
- Also produced by smooth muscle cells, activated macrophages, and ECs
- Essential in early development, tissue remodeling, differentiation
- Downstream effector pathways (MAPK, phosphatidylinositol 3-kinase [PI3K], and/or JAK/STAT) are triggered via PDGF receptor (PDGFR)A, B.

ONCOLOGIC BEHAVIORS

- *COL1A1–PDGFB* fusion linked to dermatofibrosarcoma protuberans
- PDGFRA mutations linked to multiple tumor types; germline lesions linked to hereditary gastrointestinal stromal tumors (GIST)
- *PDGFRA* amplification often associated with coalterations in epidermal growth factor receptor (*EGFR*), *KIT*, *KDR*
- Up to 60% of PDGFRA mutant GIST are also D842V, which is associated with primary resistance.

- PDGFs are potent mitogens for cells of mesenchymal origin and are synthesized, stored, and released by platelets upon activation; also produced by smooth muscle cells, activated macrophages, and ECs.
- PDGF signaling network consists of four ligands (PDGFA–D) and two transmembrane tyrosine RTKs (PDGFRα and PDGFRβ).
- These receptors transmit extracellular growth factor signaling to intracellular signaling cascades. Upon binding of the growth factor ligands, the receptors undergo dimerization and autophosphorylation of cytoplasmic kinase domains, activating the receptor.
- Downstream effects of PDGFR activation lead to differential signaling through MAPK, PI3K, and/or JAK/STAT pathways, resulting in cell proliferation, cell differentiation, survival, and migration.
- Dermatofibrosarcoma protuberans is characterized by a chromosomal translocation with formation of COL1A1–PDGFB fusion gene, causing activation of PDGFRβ in tumor cells.
- PDGFRα is encoded by the *PDGFRA* gene, which is altered in multiple tumor types, resulting in constitutive PDGFRα activity.
- Germline mutations in PDGFRA have been described in hereditary GIST.
- PDGFRA amplification has been described in sarcomas and gliomas; however, often it is associated with coalterations in EGFR, KIT, and KDR.
- In about 5% of GIST, somatic PDGFRA mutations in exons 12, 14, and 18 activation loop are the most common and are associated with greater response to PDGFRA-inhibitor imatinib. However, up to 60% of PDGFRA mutant GIST harbors a mutation in exon 18 D842V, which is associated with primary resistance.

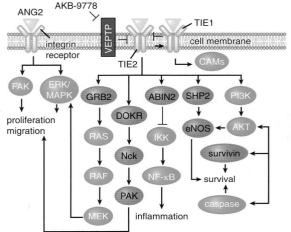

PHYSIOLOGY

- Angiopoietin growth factors (ANG) regulate angiogenesis through activating (ANG1,4) or inhibitory (ANG2,3) effects on TIE1,2.
- ANG-TIE system is critical for cardiac, blood, vascular development and homeostasis.

ASSOCIATED PATHOLOGIC STATES

- inflammation
- metastasis
- tumor angiogenesis
- atherosclerosis
- vascular leakage

ONCOGENIC BEHAVIORS

- Circulating ANG2 predictive of poor prognosis from many cancers
- Low baseline ANG2 predicts better response to anti-VEGF therapy versus colorectal cancer.
- High baseline serum ANG2 predicts poorer outcome from immune checkpoint therapy; potentially immunosuppressive.
- ANG bind to cell surface RTKs with immunoglobulin-like and epithelial growth factor–like domains 1 and 2 (TIE1 and TIE2).
- Four different ANGs have been identified (ANG1, ANG2, ANG3, and ANG4).
- ANG1 and ANG4 are agonists for TIE2, whereas ANG2 and ANG3 are competitive antagonists for TIE1 and TIE2.
- Activation of TIE2 by ANG1 is indispensable for embryonic cardiac development and angiogenesis, and both TIE1 and TIE2 are key regulators of normal formation of blood and lymphatic vessel development as TIE1 and TIE2 are almost exclusively expressed in the endothelium.
- ANG/TIE system is also involved in pathologic processes including inflammation, metastasis, tumor angiogenesis, atherosclerosis, and vascular leakage.
- Upon binding of ANG ligands, TIE2 receptors can form dimers or possibly multimers. Vascular endothelial protein tyrosine phosphatase (VEPTP, encoded by *PTPRB* gene) dephosphorylates active TIE2.
- TIE1 upregulates the cell adhesion molecules (CAMs) VCAM-1, E-selectin, and ICAM-1 through a p38-dependent mechanism.

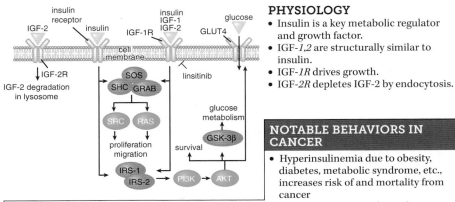

PHYSIOLOGY

- Insulin is a key metabolic regulator and growth factor.
- IGF-*1,2* are structurally similar to insulin.
- IGF-*1R* drives growth.
- IGF-*2R* depletes IGF-2 by endocytosis.

NOTABLE BEHAVIORS IN CANCER

- Hyperinsulinemia due to obesity, diabetes, metabolic syndrome, etc., increases risk of and mortality from cancer
- Glucose transporter (GLUT)4 is overexpressed in pancreatic cancers, possibly linked to castration-resistant phenotype.
- IGF-1R is overexpressed in some cancers, possibly to increase glucose uptake via insulin receptor substrate (IRS)-1-dependent membrane translocation of GLUT.
- IGF levels are prognostic in NSCLC and sarcoma.
- IGF-1R promotes resistance to EGFR drugs by dimerizing with EGFR.
- IGF-1R drugs have limited clinical activity, significant adverse effects, for example, hyperglycemia.

- Insulin-like growth factor family includes two growth factors (IGF-1, IGF-2) and two receptors (IGF-1R, IGF-2R).
- IGF-1 and IGF-2 are polypeptide hormones structurally similar to insulin. IGF-IR, IGF-2R, and insulin receptors are also structurally similar and are able to form heterodimers.
- IGF-1R is activated by IGF-1, IGF-2, and insulin and has a strong growth-promoting effect.
- IGF-2R does not trigger signaling, but regulates extracellular IRS-2 levels through receptor-mediated endocytosis and degradation. Upon phosphorylation, IGF-1R recruits and phosphorylates adaptor proteins IRS-1, IRS-2, and SRC homology 2 domain-containing protein (SHC).
- IRS-1 acts as a second messenger within cell to stimulate transcription of insulin-related genes (e.g., ELK1, glycogen synthase-3 [GSK3]) via PI3K and RAS pathways and also initiates the translocation of GLUT to the cell surface where it facilitates transport of glucose into the cell.
- IRS-2 plays a critical role in cellular motility response, and SHC stimulates activation of MAPK pathway.
- Compared with normal cells, cancer cells have an increased need for glucose, which alters cellular metabolism (i.e., Warburg effect).

- Increased levels of IGF-1R are expressed in certain types of cancer cells (e.g., prostate, pancreatic), which can lead to increased uptake of glucose from blood into tumor. However, IGF-1R expression does not consistently correlate with disease control in heterogeneous groups of patients treated with anti-IGF-1R monoclonal antibodies (mAbs).
- IGF ligand (IGF-1) levels have been shown to have predictive value in NSCLC and sarcoma, but correlation between ligand level and tumor microenvironment has not been established.
- In the presence of epidermal growth factor (EGF) inhibitors, IGF-1R can dimerize with EGFR, allowing pathway signaling to resume, leading to resistance of these inhibitors.
- Although there is compelling preclinical evidence, only limited clinical activity of IGF-1R inhibition has been observed in several tumor types, including NSCLC and breast cancer. More favorable outcomes were observed in patients with sarcoma.
- Furthermore, common adverse effects of IGF-1R inhibition that include hyperglycemia (pituitary feedback loop), nausea, vomiting, fatigue, anorexia, and skin reactions have limited the U.S. Food and Drug Administration (FDA) approval of any IGF-1R pathway inhibitors so far.

TGFα/SMAD

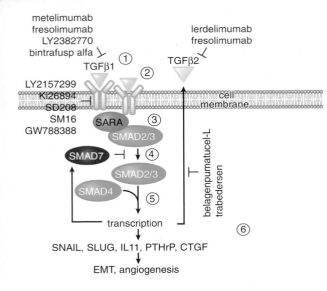

CLASSICAL SIGNALING

1. Activation of transforming growth factor-beta (TGFβ) receptors
2. Oligomerization
3. Phosphorylation of SMAD2/3
4. Translocation of SMADs to nucleus
5. Expression of target genes, for example, cyclin-dependent kinase (CDK) inhibitors
6. Physiologic response, for example, cytoskeletal rearrangement, remodeling of extracellular matrix

---

NOTABLE BEHAVIORS IN CANCER

- TGFβ is upregulated in some cancers with programmed cell death ligand 1 (PD-L1), inhibits anticancer immunity, and contributes to poor prognosis.
- SMAD4 deletion is common in pancreatic cancers, inactivating mutations in liver, colorectal cancer.
- Germline SMAD4 lesion is linked to hereditary juvenile polyposis.
- TGFβ induces tumor cell migration and boosts epithelial to mesenchymal transition.
- TGFβ is a powerful suppressor of innate and adaptive immunity, promoting immune surveillance by tumor cells.

- TGFβ signaling pathway plays a critical role in cell growth, differentiation, and development. TGFβ stimulates proliferation of mesenchymal cells, but inhibits proliferation of epithelial cells.
- In cancer, TGFβ inhibits immune response against cancer, while stimulating stromal cells to proliferate.
- Signaling is initiated by interaction of the ligand with the receptor and oligomerization of serine/threonine TGFβ receptor kinases and phosphorylation of the cytoplasmic signaling molecules SMAD2 and SMAD3.
- SMAD transcription factors are phosphorylated and translocated to nucleus where they stimulate expression of genes encoding CDK inhibitors or proteins involved in the formation and remodeling of extracellular matrix.
- Activation of pathway is counteracted by inhibitory SMADs (e.g., SMAD7), which are encoded by gene induced by pathway stimulation (feedback mechanism).
- TGFβ/activin and bone morphogenetic protein (BMP) pathways are modulated by MAPK signaling at a number of levels. Moreover, in certain contexts, TGFβ signaling can also affect

SMAD-independent pathways, including ERK, stress-activated protein kinase/c-Jun NH2-terminal kinase (SAPK/JNK), and p38 MAPK pathways.

- Rho GTPase (RhoA) activates downstream target proteins to prompt rearrangement of the cytoskeletal elements associated with cell growth, migration, and invasion.
- A germline mutation in SMAD4 is known to be associated with hereditary juvenile polyposis syndrome.
- Targeting TGFβ can be done by different drugs that include antisense oligonucleotides (AONs), neutralizing antibodies that inhibit ligand–receptor interactions, receptor domain–immunoglobulin fusions that sequester ligands and prevent binding to receptors, and receptor kinase inhibitors.
  - AONs (target TGFβ2): trabedersen (AP12009) and antisense gene-modified allogenic tumor vaccine: Belagenpumatucel-L (Lucanix) are currently in clinical trials.
  - Antibodies: Fresolimumab (GC-1008)—binds TGFβ1 and TGFβ2; IMC-TR1—targets TβRII
  - TGFβ kinase inhibitors/small-molecule inhibitors: LY2157299 (galunisertib); TEW-7197
- Although TGFβ targeting agents, such as galunisertib, have shown dramatic therapeutic effects in animal cancer models and in some cancer patients, it is still not clear how the therapeutic effect in cancer patients is achieved; currently, there is no predictive biomarker for response to drugs targeting the TGFβ pathway.
- TGFβ and PD-L1 are both upregulated in certain types of cancers, and their overexpression is associated with increased evasion of immune surveillance and contributes to poor prognosis.
- Bintrafusp alfa, a bifunctional fusion protein composed of avelumab, an anti-PD-L1 human mAb, bound to the soluble extracellular domain of TGFβRII, has shown to increase natural killer (NK) cell and cytotoxic T-lymphocyte (CTL) activities inhibiting tumor cell proliferation; it is currently being tested in clinical trials.

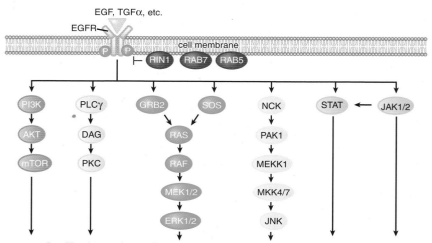

EGF, TGFα, etc.

EGFR

cell membrane

RIN1 RAB7 RAB5

PI3K PLCγ GRB2 SOS NCK STAT JAK1/2

AKT DAG RAS PAK1

mTOR PKC RAF MEKK1

MEK1/2 MKK4/7

ERK1/2 JNK

cell proliferation, angiogenesis, migration, adhesion, inhibition of apoptosis, invasion

PHYSIOLOGY
- Family consists of EGFR (ERBB1), HER2 (ERBB2), HER3 (ERBB3), HER4 (ERBB4).
- EGFR, HER2, HER4 are active kinases.

EGF FAMILY OF RECEPTORS
- The EGF family of receptors are transmembrane RTKs that are frequently overexpressed or mutated in a wide variety of epithelial tumors.
- The EGF or ERBB family consists of EGFR (ERBB1), HER2 (ERBB2), HER3 (ERBB3), and HER4 (ERBB4).
- They are characterized by an extracellular ligand-binding domain and an intracellular tyrosine kinase domain except ERBB3, which has a kinase-deficient intracellular domain.

ACTIVATION OF THE RECEPTORS
- The EGF family of receptors is activated by binding to a ligand resulting in homo- or heterodimerization of the receptors and phosphorylation of the receptors at the cytosolic kinase domain. This results in the recruitment of adapter molecules, leading to activation of signaling pathway cascades downstream.
- One of the well-studied pathways acts through the RAS → rapidly accelerated fibrosarcoma (RAF) → ERK cascade. The other major pathway involves the lipid kinase PI3K, AKT, and mammalian target of rapamycin (mTOR). The activation of these pathways leads to cell growth, proliferation, differentiation, and migration.
- The receptor is trafficked through the early and late endosomes and lysosomes, where it is degraded by proteases. This regulation mechanism driven by RAB5, RIN1, and RAB7 ensures downregulation of receptor signaling when not required.

LIGANDS
- EGFR (ERBB1) has seven known ligands: EGF, TGFα, heparin-binding EGF-like growth factor (HBEGF), amphiregulin (AREG), β-cellulin (BTC), epiregulin (EREG), and epigen (EPGN). EGF and TGFα are the most common and most characterized.

- Interestingly, ERBB2 (HER2) does not have a ligand. ERBB2 can heterodimerize with EGFR, ERBB3, and ERBB4, functioning through activation of other receptor family members.
- Neuregulin 1 and 2 bind ERBB3 to activate it, whereas EGF, BTC, and neuregulins (1–4) bind ERBB4.

EGFR SIGNALING IN CANCER

- Dysregulation of EGFR signaling is seen in cancer.
- EGFR kinase domain mutations are commonly seen in lung cancer. These result in constitutive activation of the EGF receptor.
- EGFR overexpression is commonly seen in head and neck squamous cell carcinoma (80%–90%), NSCLC (~60%), triple-negative breast cancer (~60%), colon cancer (>90%), and glioblastoma (~50%). EGFR overexpression can occur by increase in copy number or increase in protein expression.
- Other mechanisms of signaling dysregulation include defective downregulation of the receptor (caused by CBL mutations and seen in EGFRvIII) and cross-talk with other receptors (such as other ERBB family members and G-protein-coupled receptors or GPCRs).

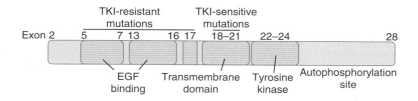

Notable behaviors in cancer	• Overexpressed in head and neck squamous cell carcinoma (80%–90%), NSCLC (~60%), triple-negative breast cancer (~60%), colon cancer (>90%), and glioblastoma (~50%). • Constitutively active mutants common in lung cancer • Normal switch-off mechanisms may be lost • May cross-talk with other receptors	
EGFR-activating mutations	• L858R on exon 21 • in-frame deletion in exon 19	• Account for 90% of activating mutations
	• L861Q (exon 21) • G719X (exon 18) • V765A, T783A (exon 20) • Some in-frame deletion/insertion on exon 20 • T790M: most common lesion that confers resistance to EGFR drugs	
EGFR VIII	• Truncated form after deletion of exons 2–7 by gene rearrangement • Unable to bind ligand, but is constitutively active because of interaction with wild-type EGFR and loss of downregulation mechanism • Preferentially triggers PI3K/AKT, whereas other mutants activate MAPK	

Activating mutations, except exon 20 insertions, hypersensitize cells to EGFR inhibitors. Exon 20 mutations contribute to resistance to EGFR inhibitors.

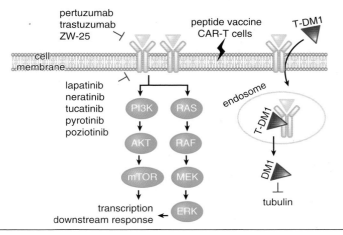

NOTABLE BEHAVIORS IN CANCER

- Overexpression, rather than simple activation, is required for tumorigenic activity.
- Overexpression may alter the repertoire of HER2-containing dimers, resulting in altered signaling.
- Overexpression deregulates cell cycle, polarity, and adhesion.
- Overexpression elicits oncogene addiction, the basis of drug activity.

LESIONS IN CANCER

- Overexpressed/amplified in breast (~30% of tumors), esophageal (~17%), lung (~3%), ovarian (~2%–66%), colorectal (~3%), prostate, salivary gland, bladder cancer
- In-frame A775_G776insYVMA in exon 20 seen in NSCLC
- Activating missense mutations in kinase domain seen in breast, lung, colorectal cancers
- Activating mutations in extracellular domain, for example, S310Y and S310F, are seen in ~1%–2% lung and breast cancers, some colorectal and ovarian cancers.

- HER2 (ERBB2) is the second member of the EGFR family of receptors.
- HER2 heterodimerizes with EGFR as well as ERBB3.
- ERBB2/HER2 is often overexpressed/amplified in various cancer types such as breast (~30% of tumors), esophageal (~17% of tumors), lung (~3%), ovarian (~2%–66%), colorectal cancer (~3%). Amplification is also seen in prostate cancer, salivary gland tumors, and bladder cancers.
- *ERBB2* gene mutations are drivers of several cancer types. In NSCLC, ERBB2 exon 20 in-frame insertion/duplication A775_G776insYVMA is the most prevalent.
- Missense activating mutations in tyrosine kinase domains are seen in breast, lung, and colorectal cancers predominantly.
- Extracellular domain mutations causing enhanced kinase activity such as ERBB2 S310Y and ERBB2 S310F are seen in ~1% to 2% lung and breast cancers, and also a small proportion of colorectal and ovarian cancers.

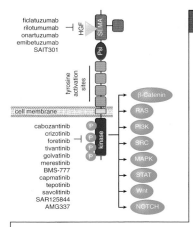

NOTABLE BEHAVIORS IN CANCER

- Deregulation linked to tumor growth, metastasis, poor prognosis
- Hepatocyte growth factor (HGF) lesions linked to kidney, liver, gastric, esophageal, breast, brain, and melanoma
- Cancer stem cells seem to reacquire MET expression, which is normally exclusive to stem and progenitor cells.
- MET activation synergizes with INK4a/alternate reading frame (ARF) inactivation in rhabdomyosarcoma.
- MET amplification and exon 14 skipping drive NSCLC progression and resistance to EGFR drugs.
- MET amplification linked to aggressive gastric cancer and poor outcome
- Tumor HGF secretion drives MET expression in melanoma.

- Constitutive activation of the HGF promoter is observed in 51% of African-Americans with breast cancer.
- Circulating HGF levels correlated with poorer survival and are potential markers for both presence of cancer and disease stage.

NORMAL BIOLOGY

- c-MET is a proto-oncogene that encodes for hepatocyte growth factor receptor, also known as MET (HGFR), possessing tyrosine kinase activity.
- HGF is the only known ligand of the MET receptor.
- MET induces several biologic responses that collectively give rise to invasive growth.

ROLE IN CANCER

- Abnormal MET activation in cancer correlates with poor prognosis, where uncontrolled MET triggers tumor growth, angiogenesis, and metastasis.
- MET deregulation (MET and HGF amplifications, MET mutations) has been implicated in many types of cancer, including kidney, liver, gastric, esophageal, breast, brain, and melanoma.
- Usually, only stem cells and progenitor cells express MET, which allows for invasive growth; however, cancer stem cells are thought to hijack the ability of normal stem cells to express MET and thus become the cause of cancer persistence and metastasis.
- MET activates multiple signal transduction pathways, including RAS, PI3K, STAT, Wnt, and NOTCH.
- Inactivation of tumor suppressors INK4a/ARF synergizes with MET activation in rhabdomyosarcoma.
- MET expression is driven by HGF secretions in the tumor cell microenvironment in melanoma.
- In NSCLC, c-MET amplification and exon 14 skipping drive progression and resistance to EGFR inhibitors. In gastric cancers, amplification is associated with aggressive disease and poor outcomes.

Physiology	• Receptor for glial cell line–derived neurotropic factors (GDNF) • Activates MAPK and PI3K pathways similar to EGFR.
Notable behaviors in cancer	• Point mutations drive multiple endocrine neoplasia syndromes (MEN2) and familial medullary thyroid cancer. • Fusion with other proteins may cause constitutive activation, potentially via dimerization. • Fusions associated with radiation exposure, seen in NSCLC, Spitz tumors, breast, colon cancers, ~1/3 of papillary thyroid cancers • Fusion partners include KIF5B, CCDC6, GOLGA5, TRIM24, TRIM27, TRIM33, PRKAR1A, MBD1, KTN1, HOOK3, AKAP13, FKBP15, SPECC1L, ERC1, NCOA4, TBL1XR1, RAB6IP2

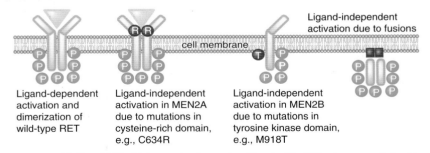

Ligand-dependent activation and dimerization of wild-type RET

Ligand-independent activation in MEN2A due to mutations in cysteine-rich domain, e.g., C634R

Ligand-independent activation in MEN2B due to mutations in tyrosine kinase domain, e.g., M918T

Ligand-independent activation due to fusions

(Adapted from Romei C, Ciampi R, Elisei R. A comprehensive overview of the role of the RET proto-oncogene in thyroid carcinoma. *Nat Rev Endocrinol.* 2016;12(4):192–202.)

- REarranged during Transfection (RET) receptor can activate MAPK and PI3K pathways similar to EGFR.
- RET is a receptor for the GDNF family of extracellular ligands.

ROLE IN CANCER

- Point mutations in RET give rise to MEN2 and familial medullary thyroid cancer.
- Chromosomal rearrangements that create a fusion between RET and other proteins can cause constitutive activation of RET receptor.
- Fusions of RET with other genes have been identified in multiple malignancies.
  - Found in approximately one-third of patients with papillary thyroid cancer. Associated with radiation exposure.
  - RET fusions have also been identified as an oncogenic driver in NSCLC, Spitz tumors, breast, and colon cancers.
  - RET fusion partners include KIF5B, CCDC6, GOLGA5, TRIM24, TRIM27, TRIM33, PRKAR1A, MBD1, KTN1, HOOK3, AKAP13, FKBP15, SPECC1L, ERC1, NCOA4, TBL1XR1, and RAB6IP2. Many of these partners have dimerization motifs, suggesting this as a possible mechanism for RET activation.

Physiology	• Also known as CD246; receptor for insulin • Expressed in brain, testis, small intestine; enhanced expression in developing nervous system; lower expression in adults
Notable behaviors in cancer	• Overactivated following fusion with other genes, typically via constitutive dimerization • Amplification and gene deletions seen in several malignancies, e.g., in 13 of 15 specimens of inflammatory breast cancer • Nonfusion lesions of unknown significance, although mutation and overexpression seen in 40%–100% of neuroblastomas

NOTABLE FUSIONS

Physiology	Partners	Prev. (%)
Lymphoma	NPM, TPM3, TPM4	60
NSCLC	EML4, K1F5B	5
Colorectal	EML4	2
Breast	EML4	2
Renal	EML4, TPM3	2

• **NPM binds ss- and dsDNA; drives DNA repair, stabilizes genome**
• **TPM3 drives muscle contraction**
• **EML4 modifies microtubules**
• **K1F5B required to distribute mitochondria, lysosomes**

ROLE IN CANCER

- Observed mechanisms of oncogenesis involve overactivation of the ALK receptor through fusion gene formation. The most common is the EML4–ALK fusion, occurring in 2% to 7% of NSCLCs.
- ALK fusions were first discovered in lymphoma. In solid tumors, they are found most commonly in lung adenocarcinoma, but have been identified in Spitz tumors, sarcoma, melanoma, breast, colorectal, esophageal, cholangiocarcinoma, thyroid, neuroblastoma, renal cell, renal medullary, and bladder cancers.
- Fusion partner usually has a domain that induces constitutive dimerization with resultant activation.
- In NSCLC, patients with ALK fusions are usually young with minimal or no smoking history.
- ALK amplifications and gene deletions have been identified in several malignancies. At this time, the significance of nonfusion alterations is unclear.
- Crizotinib was the first-generation ALK inhibitor; second-generation inhibitors include ceritinib, alectinib, and brigatinib; lorlatinib is a third-generation inhibitor.

Physiology	• Regulates cell survival, proliferation, differentiation • Expressed as multiple transcript variants encoding isoforms • Strongly expressed by hematopoietic stem cells, multipotent progenitors, common myeloid progenitors, early thymocyte progenitors; lower levels of expression in common lymphoid progenitors, mast cells, melanocytes, interstitial cells of Cajal in digestive tract
Lesions in Cancer	• Activating mutations linked to GIST, testicular seminoma, mast cell disease, melanoma, acute myeloid leukemia • Primary mutations in exon 11 and 9 linked to sensitivity and intrinsic resistance to imatinib, respectively • Secondary mutations in kinase domain (exons 13–18) linked to acquired resistance to imatinib.

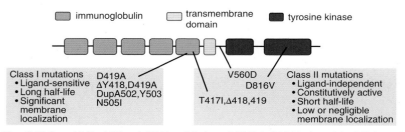

(Adapted from Shi X, Sousa LP, Mandel-Bausch EM, Tome F, Reshetnyak AV, Hadari Y, Schlessinger J, Lax I. Distinct cellular properties of oncogenic KIT receptor tyrosine kinase mutants enable alternative courses of cancer cell inhibition. *Proc Natl Acad Sci U S A.* 2016;113(33):E4784–E4793.)

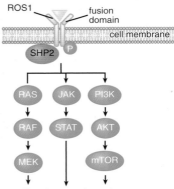

Physiology

- Structurally similar to ALK, but activated by unknown ligand
- Function also unknown, but contains extracellular sequences analogous to cell adhesion proteins, triggers typical RTK pathways
- In normal adults, expression is highest in the kidney, with some expression in stomach, intestines, neural tissue.

Lesions in Cancer

- Fusion with various partners enhances oncogenesis.
- ROS-1 rearrangement relatively rare, seen only in the absence of other known oncogenic driver mutations
- ROS-1 mutation seen in ~2% of NSCLCs

Fusion partners		
TPM3	CD74	KDELR2
CEP85L	TFG	ZER
CCDC6	FIG	YWHAE
SLC34A2	SDC4	LRIG3

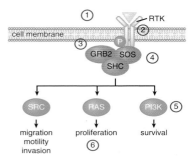

Signaling

1. Activation by growth factors
2. Homo- or heterodimerization
3. Autophosphorylation
4. Recruitment of adaptor proteins
5. Activation of downstream pathways
6. Physiologic response

Oncogenic Mechanisms

- **Activating gain-of-function mutations**
- **Overexpression because of genomic amplification**

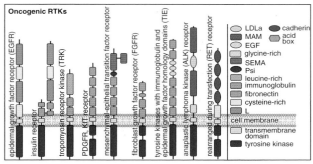

- RTKs are cell surface receptors that function as key regulators of fundamental cellular processes such as proliferation, differentiation, senescence, and migration, among others.
- Binding growth factor ligands to extracellular domain, RTKs induce receptor dimerization (forming either homodimers or heterodimers with other RTKs) followed by their autophosphorylation. This allows for subsequent recruitment of adaptor proteins such as growth factor receptor–bound protein 2 (GRB2), SHC, and Son of Sevenless (SOS) that activate proliferation, survival, and migration pathways (e.g., RAS, PI3K, SRC).
- Tight control of RTK activation is necessary for tissue homeostasis, which is why RTKs constitute one of the biggest classes of oncoproteins.
- Over 20 different classes of RTKs have been identified, including the following that have been previously implicated in cancer initiation and progression: ALK, EGFR, FGFR, IGFR, KIT, MET, PDGFR, RET, TIE, and VEGFR. Each RTK will be discussed in detail in this section.

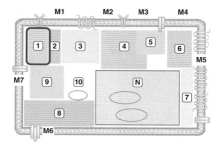

Rapamycin is a naturally occurring "antibiotic" discovered on the Pacific island of Rapa Nui (Easter Island) in the 1970s. This "family" consists of the mTOR complex, PI3K, AKT, phosphatase and tensin homolog (PTEN) and is an important key regulator of the immune system, glucose metabolism, and cell growth.

PI3K activation leads to phosphorylation and activation of AKT, which in turn can activate mTOR. The pathway can be suppressed by tuberous sclerosis (TSC1; hamartin), TSC2 (tuberin), and phosphatidylinositol-3,4,5-trisphosphate 3-phosphatase (PTEN). PI3Ks are divided into three classes according to structural characteristics and substrate specificity. This pathway interacts with IRS to regulate glucose uptake through a series of phosphorylation events. Hyperglycemia and sore mouth are common but manageable side effects in patients taking PI3K inhibitors.

Easter Island is a triangular-shaped Chilean territory in the Pacific Ocean and is known for the remarkable stone head sculptures.

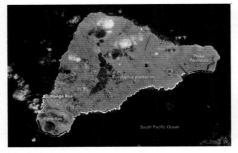

(NASA Earth Observatory image by Jesse Allen, using Landsat data from the U.S. Geological Survey. Available at https://earthobservatory.nasa.gov/images/90027/easter-island)

(From Shutterstock.)

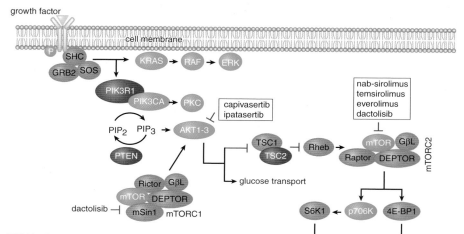

PI3K classes

Class IA	Catalytic	PIK3CA,B,D
	Regulatory	PI3KR1,2,3
Class II	Catalytic	PIK3C2A,2B,2G

Class IB	Catalytic	PIK3CG
	Regulatory	PI3KR5
Class III	Catalytic	PIK3C3

- PI3K/protein kinase B (PKB or AKT)/mTOR pathway is a key regulator of normal cellular processes. Aberrant activation of this pathway leads to survival and proliferation of tumor cells.
- PI3K activation leads to phosphorylation and activation of AKT, which in turn can activate mTOR. The pathway can be suppressed by TSC1 (hamartin), TSC2 (tuberin), and PTEN.
- PI3Ks are divided into three classes according to structural characteristics and substrate specificity:
  - Class I
    - Class IA PI3Ks: heterodimers consisting of a p110 catalytic subunit (isoforms p110α, p110β, and p110δ encoded by the genes *PIK3CA*, *PIK3CB*, and *PIK3CD*, respectively) and a p85 regulatory subunit (isoforms p85α [and slice variants p55α and p50α] encoded by PIK3R1, p85β encoded by PIK3R2, and p85γ encoded by PIK3R3)
    - Class IB PI3Ks: heterodimers consisting of a p110γ (encoded by PIK3CG) and a p101 regulatory subunit (encoded by PIK3R5)
  - Class II: monomers with a single catalytic subunit (isoforms PI3KC2α, PI3KC2β, and PI3KC2γ encoded by PIK3C2A, PIK3C2B, and PIK3C2G, respectively)
  - Class III: single catalytic subunit VPS34 (encoded by *PIK3C3* gene)
- This pathway interacts with the IRS to regulate glucose uptake through a series of phosphorylation events. A common side effect in patients taking PI3Ks inhibitors is hyperglycemia.

Molecule	Notable Behaviors in Cancer
PIK3CA	Activating missense mutations occur throughout, with most in hotspots, e.g., E542K, E545K in exon 9; H1047R in exon 20
PIK3R1	• Substitutions, in-frame insertions, deletions in iSH2 domain that impair inhibitory activity against catalytic subunit • Somatic mutations prevalent in endometrial, glioma, colon cancer • Suppressed in some cancers
PIK3CB	Seen in breast and castration-resistant prostate cancer
PIK3CD PIK3CG	Typically not mutated, but amplified or overexpressed
PIK3R2	• Somatic mutations in endometrial, colorectal cancer, but no hotspot • Overexpression in breast, colon cancer
PIK3C2B	• Like PIK3C2A, expressed in tumor cells • Mutations seen in NSCLC • Amplification in glioblastoma
AKT1	• E17K in melanoma, breast, colorectal, endometrial, ovarian, squamous cell lung cancer; amplification in gastric cancer
AKT2	• Mutations in colorectal cancer; amplification in head and neck, pancreatic, ovarian, breast cancers
AKT3	• Amplification in melanoma, breast, endometrial, ovarian cancer
PTEN	• Germline mutations linked to inherited PTEN hamartoma tumor syndrome (PHTS) that increase the risk of breast, thyroid, endometrial cancer
TSC1/2	• Mutations linked to bladder, kidney cancers

TARGETING AKT MUTATIONS

- AKT (also known as PKB) is a serine–threonine protein kinase expressed as three isoforms AKT1, AKT2, and AKT3 (encoded by the genes *PKBα*, *PKBβ*, and *PKBγ*, respectively).
- Activation through mutation has been reported for all three isoforms (AKT1, AKT2, AKT3) and activation through amplification has been reported for two isoforms only (AKT1, AKT2). They affect survival, proliferation, and apoptosis of cancer cells with additional effects on tumor-induced angiogenesis through activation of other kinases (e.g., BCL-2-associated death promoter [BAD], mouse double minute 2 [MDM2], GSK3β).
  - AKT1 is involved in cell survival and growth.
    - Mutation E17K in AKT1 has been identified in melanoma, breast, colorectal, endometrial, and ovarian cancers.
    - Mutation is most common in breast, colorectal, and squamous cell lung carcinoma cancers; amplification is most common in gastric cancer.
  - AKT2 is involved in invasiveness and insulin responsiveness.
    - Mutation is most common in colorectal cancer; amplification is common in head and neck, pancreatic, ovary, and breast cancers.
  - AKT3 is involved in survival and apoptosis.
    - Amplification is common in a wide variety of cancers, for example, breast, endometrial, ovarian, and melanoma.

TARGETING PTEN AND TSC ALTERATIONS

- PTEN is a lipid phosphatase that removes phosphate on the three positions of PIP3 and converts it back to PIP2.
- Germline mutations in the *PTEN* gene are associated with inherited cancer predisposition syndromes collectively known as PHTS (e.g., Cowden syndrome and Bannayan–Riley–Ruvalcaba syndrome); individuals with PHTS have an increased incidence of breast, thyroid, and endometrial cancers.
- Preclinical data suggest mTOR inhibitors exhibit activity against PTEN alterations.
- TSC1 or hamartin and TSC2 or tuberin proteins are tumor suppressors in the PI3K pathway.
- TSC1–TSC2 (hamartin–tuberin) complex is a critical negative regulator of mTORC1 through its GAP (GTPase-activating protein) activity toward the small G-protein Rheb (Ras homolog enriched in brain).
- Germline TSC1/2 mutations have been linked to bladder and kidney cancers.
- Loss of TSC1/2 function leads to overactivity of mTOR; therefore, mTOR inhibitors may show activity against TSC alterations.

mTORC1,2

PHYSIOLOGY

- Considered to be class IV PI3Ks
- Activated in response to growth factors and nutrients
- A master regulator of metabolic homeostasis, protein and lipid synthesis, glycolysis, mitochondria biogenesis, lysosome biogenesis, proteasome assembly, and autophagy

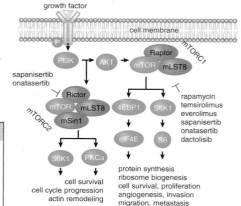

NOTABLE BEHAVIORS IN CANCER

- Mutations (potentially hyperactivating, usually rapamycin-sensitive) detected in colorectal, endometrial, lung cancers
- Amplification of other subunits, for example, raptor, has been seen.
- Also activated by oncogenic activation of upstream regulators, for example, RTKs, PI3K
- Mediates metabolic reprogramming to ensure tumor cell survival and proliferation; also responds to upstream metabolic changes, for example, increased glucose or amino acid uptake
- mTORC inhibitors are being tested in combination with other drugs that interfere with cellular metabolism, for example, the diabetes drug metformin.

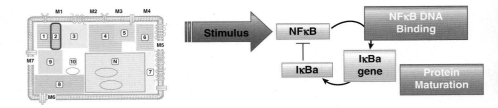

Nuclear factor kappa B (NF-κB) is an ancient protein transcription factor and considered a regulator of innate immunity. The NF-κB signaling pathway links pathogenic signals and cellular danger signals, thus organizing cellular resistance to invading pathogens.

NF-κB is a network hub responsible for complex biologic signaling and is considered a master regulator of evolutionarily conserved biochemical cascades. Other factors are also translocated into the mitochondria and are involved in modulating expression.

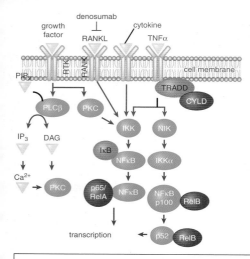

NOTABLE BEHAVIORS IN CANCER

- Osteoclasts, which express RANK, are aberrantly activated in metastatic bone cancer.
- NF-κB links chronic inflammation to cancer.
- NF-κB lesions are typical in lymphoid cancers, rarer in solid cancers.
- NF-κB may be constitutively activated by lesions in upstream regulators or by deregulated secretion of cytokines and other stimuli.
- Constitutive NF-κB activation elicits chemo- and radio-resistance.
- Depending on context, NF-κB can trigger or suppress tumorigenesis.

PHYSIOLOGY

- Cytokine receptors triggered by interferons (e.g., IFNα,β,γ); interleukins (e.g., IL-2)
- RANKL expressed on stromal cells, osteoblasts, T cells
- RANK expressed on osteoclasts, dendritic cells; regulates immune signaling

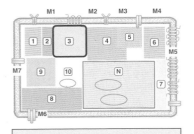

Nobel Prizes in 1994 and 2012

GPCRs are "seven-transmembrane" globular proteins that make up the largest and most diverse group of cell surface receptors. They are named for their binding to guanosine diphosphate (GDP). The conversion of GDP to the triphosphate GTP is the "on/off" switch that positively (+) or negatively (−) affects hundreds of "druggable" enzyme cascades.

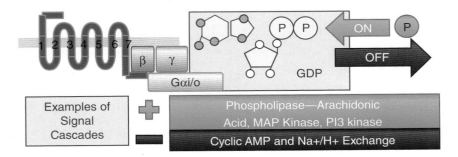

Examples of Signal Cascades

+ Phospholipase—Arachidonic Acid, MAP Kinase, PI3 kinase

− Cyclic AMP and Na+/H+ Exchange

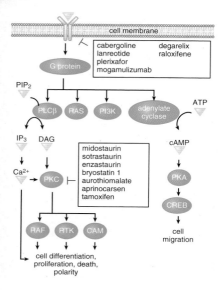

PHYSIOLOGY

- Large family of receptors that regulate multiple signaling pathways
- Activated by diverse ligands, for example, chemokines, hormones, neurotransmitters
- Targeted by the most successful drugs to manage pain, inflammation, neurologic, and metabolic disorders

NOTABLE BEHAVIORS IN CANCER

- Downstream effector PKC frequently dysregulated in cancers
- Deregulated levels of GPCR ligands in the circulation or tumor environment trigger sustained activation, driving tumor growth
- GPCR mutations seen in ~20% of cancers; constitutively active G-protein mutants may drive carcinogenesis.

EMERGING TARGETS OF ANTICANCER DRUGS

- Chemokine, lysophospholipid receptors
- Protease-activated, E-prostanoid receptors
- Smoothened (SMO), Frizzled (FZD) receptors
- GPCRs that regulate Hippo, "transactivate" RTKs

Mitogen-Activated Protein Kinase (MAPK)

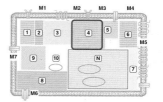

Since the 1980s, the MAP kinases have been an important source of cell signal research. They are specific to the amino acids serine and threonine and control responses to cellular stress: mitogens, heat shock, and inflammatory cytokines. MAPK/ERK regulates cell proliferation, differentiation, mitosis, and apoptosis.

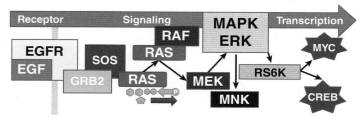

The MAPK "Cascade": Epidermal Growth Factor Receptor (**EGFR**); Growth factor receptor–bound protein 2 (**GRB2**); Son of Sevenless (**SOS**); **RAS** (RAt Sarcoma virus), a small GTPase that is related to G proteins. Rapidly Accelerated Fibrosarcoma (**RAF**); **MEK** is the MAP Kinase Kinase that activates MAPK/ERK. MNKs are downstream effector kinases; RS6K is Ribosomal S6 Kinase; MYK is named for MYeloCytomatosis avian virus. CREB is Cyclic AMP Response Element–Binding Protein.

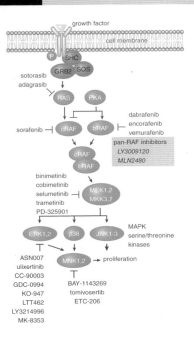

NOTABLE BEHAVIORS IN CANCER

- Sustained pathway signaling following oncogenic activation
- RAS mutations present in up to 30% of cancers
- Constitutively active KRAS (mutated in codons 12, 13, and 61) frequent in pancreatic, colon, lung cancer; KRAS mutations most common Ras lesions (25%–30%)
- HRAS mutations most frequent in bladder cancer, seminoma, Hurthle cell carcinoma
- NRAS mutations common in leukemia, melanoma, thyroid, rectal, follicular cancers
- CRAF overexpressed in lung, liver, prostate, neuroendocrine, myeloid leukemia
- BRAF seen in melanoma (30%–60%), thyroid cancer (30%–50%), colorectal cancer (5%–20%), of which 905 is V600E.
- MEK1/2 mutation and BRAF amplification in V600E cancers may confer resistance to MEK drugs.

- Signaling through the RAS/RAF/MEK/ERK (MAPK) pathway is essential for the proliferation of normal cells as well as for many cancer cells.
- Activation of pathway occurs through growth factor binding to RTKs and also by other extra- and intracellular stimuli.
- MAPK are involved in directing cellular responses to a variety of stimuli and help regulate proliferation, gene expression, and apoptosis, among others.
- In cancer cells, pathway signaling is often heightened as a consequence of oncogenic activation of RTKs, RAS, or RAF. The pathway cascade ultimately leads to ERK activation.
- MAPK kinases activated by MEK1/2 were previously known as ERK1 and ERK2 (extracellular signal–regulated kinases). MAPKs are serine/threonine kinases that include ERK1/2, P38 kinase, ERK5, and c-Jun (JNK1/2/3) kinases.

TARGETING BRAF

- RAF kinase family is serine/threonine-specific protein kinases that mediate signal transduction in MAPK pathway. Raf kinase family consists of three isoforms: RAF-1/CRAF, BRAF, ARAF.
- All Raf proteins share MEK1/2 kinases as a substrate.
- CRAF overexpression is found in a variety of primary human cancers: lung, liver, prostate, neuroendocrine tumors, and myeloid leukemia.
- BRAF mutations are found in melanoma (30%–60%), thyroid cancer (30%–50%), colorectal cancer (5%–20%).
- The most common BRAF mutation, valine (V) is substituted for by glutamate (E) at codon 600 (now referred to as V600E) in the activation segment, which accounts for 90% of BRAF mutations that are seen in human cancers. BRAF V600E mutation indicates poor prognosis in colorectal cancers.

TARGETING KRAS

- Specific KRASG12C inhibitors are now approved or in clinical trials, e.g., sotorasib and adagrasib.
- KRASG12D or pan-RAS inhibitors are upcoming.

TARGETING MEK

- MAP kinase kinases or MAPKK (also known as MEK or MAP2K) is a family of kinase enzymes in the RAS MAPK pathway.
- Inhibitors of MEK1/2 have shown efficacy in BRAF- and KRAS-mutated cancers.
- Mutations in MEK1/2 and BRAF amplification have been identified as potential mechanisms of resistance to MEK inhibitors in cancer cells harboring BRAF V600E mutation.

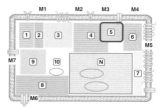

Peyton Rous discovered Rous sarcoma virus (RSV) in the early 1900s working with naturally occurring tumors in chickens. He found that by injecting RSV as a cell filtrate, RSV could induce solid tumors in closely related healthy fowl. He was awarded the Nobel Prize in 1966 for the discovery that viruses could cause tumors and cancer.

The genetic material of RSV—RSV is derived from the more common avian leukosis virus (ALV)—is ribonucleic acid (RNA), which can be transcribed into DNA by reverse transcriptase. Once incorporated into host DNA, proto-oncogene cellular c-Src function increases. Src is a nine-member family of nonreceptor tyrosine kinases. Src triggers downstream phosphorylation signaling and is linked to cancer promotion and carcinogenesis. Bishop and Varmus were awarded the Nobel Prize in 1989 for their work that included the startling discovery that one Src gene is normally present in virtually all animals and is "hijacked" as part of the process of carcinogenesis.

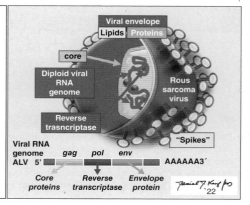

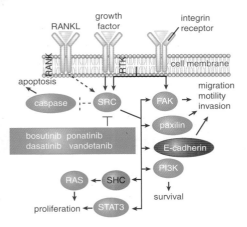

PHYSIOLOGY

- SRC is a nonreceptor tyrosine kinase that triggers phosphorylation cascades.
- Integrins mediate cell–matrix interactions, attachment of actin cytoskeleton at focal adhesion sites.
- May trigger or protect cells from apoptosis
- SRC may also act as direct effector of G proteins, and thus of GPCRs.

NOTABLE BEHAVIORS IN CANCER

- Pathway activated in ~50% of colon, liver, lung, breast, pancreatic tumors
- SRC usually overexpressed/overactive but not mutated, although mutations have been seen in colon cancer
- Activation linked to epithelial–mesenchymal transition, malignant transformation, and, subsequently, heavy migration of and invasion by cancer cells

- E-cadherin mutations seen in gastric, prostate cancers
- Altered integrin expression enables metastasis.
- SRC may also control tumor angiogenesis.
- SRC (short for sarcoma) is a family of nonreceptor protein tyrosine kinases that play an important role in the regulation of cell adhesion, invasion, and motility by phosphorylating specific tyrosine residues in other proteins such as RAS, CAMs (e.g., FAK, focal adhesion protein), and cadherins (e.g., E-cadherins).
- FAK activation by SRC is particularly important for cell adhesion and motility that leads to metastasis.
- SRC activates RAS pathway via SHC.
- SRC also activates E-cadherin, a tumor suppressor that regulates cell invasion.
- Activation of pathway is observed in approximately 50% tumors from colon, liver, lung, breast, and pancreas.
- SRC kinases are usually overexpressed or overactive in cancers, but not mutated, although mutations have been identified (e.g., colon cancer).
  - Activation is often associated with advanced stages of cancer, where cells become highly invasive and migratory.
  - Mutations in E-cadherin have been identified in gastric and prostate cancers.
- SRC is activated by RTK, integrin, VEGFR, and RANK/tumor necrosis factor (TNF)-11.
- Integrin receptors are a family of more than 24 heterodimers that mediate interactions between extracellular matrix and cells and also intracellular signal transduction.
- Altered integrin receptor expression in cancer cells can enable the mobility of metastasizing cells.
- Integrins mediate cell–matrix interactions by binding to extracellular matrix.
- Provide a focus to organize attachment of actin cytoskeleton at focal adhesion contacts

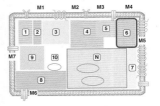

Rolf Kemler et al. (late 1980s) isolated β-catenin and two other molecules, associated with cell adhesion (E-cadherin).

Wnt (**W**ingless fruit fly **Int**egrated) proteins bind to FZD membrane seven-pass receptors. β-Catenin (Axin, Dsh, APC, GSK3, casein kinase-1 [CK1]) is phosphorylated and targeted in the "off state" and for degradation. FZD inhibits phosphorylation and β-catenin accumulates in the nucleus, binds to T-cell factors (TCF), and regulates the cell cycle.

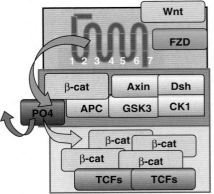

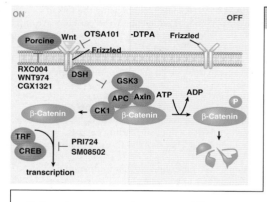

PHYSIOLOGY

- Pivotal in cell proliferation, differentiation, growth, survival, development, regeneration, homeostasis
- Regulates stemness, including of cancer stem cells; can induce dedifferentiation of intestinal epithelial cells into stem cells
- Controls proliferation, maturation, and differentiation of T cells and dendritic cells
- Deregulation drives cancer, metabolic disorders, degenerative diseases

- β-Catenin overexpression, impaired β-catenin degradation, overexpression of Wnt ligands seen in cancer cells
- Persistent signaling because of loss of APC is a key driver of colorectal cancer.
- Wnt signaling activated in 50% of breast cancers and linked to poorer overall survival

- Wnt signaling delays senescence because of BRAFV^{600E} or NRAS^{Q61K}, increasing the risk of developing melanoma; mediates phenotypic switching in melanomas between proliferative and invasive states.
- The Wnt signaling pathway is pivotal in cell proliferation, differentiation, growth, survival, development, regeneration, and homeostasis.
- Signaling is initiated by binding of the Wnt proteins to their seven-pass transmembrane receptors called FZD, which then activates β-catenin.
- In the absence of the ligand, the Wnt pathway is in an "off" state with β-catenin phosphorylated and targeted for degradation. In the "on" state, however, FZD is activated by ligand binding, which then inhibits phosphorylation and results in the translocation of β-catenin to the nucleus.
- β-Catenin initiates the transcription of its target gene with a nuclear binding partner, transcription factors of the TCF/lymphoid enhancer factor (Lef) family. These regulate the cell cycle including c-myc and CCND1.
- Porcupine protein (PORCN), located in the endoplasmic reticulum (ER), is important for processing Wnt ligand secretion.
- Deregulation of Wnt signaling contributes to the disease states such as cancer, metabolic diseases, and also degenerative diseases. Thus, inhibitors of this pathway could be used to reverse the pathologic state.
- Dysregulation of the pathway in cancer cells may be associated with mutations in β-catenin that result in overexpression, deficiencies in β-catenin destruction complex, and overexpression of Wnt ligands.
- Small-molecule inhibitors have been used to target the Wnt signaling pathway by targeting cytoplasmic proteins, transcription factors, and/or other coactivators.

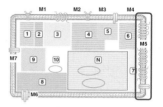

In 1933, Thomas Morgan Hunt received the Nobel Prize for research on *Drosophila melanogaster*—fruit fly genes (FFG). Many of these genes are also fundamental to normal human development because they are mutated and "hijacked" in the process of carcinogenesis. Mutated FFGs are important new drug targets.

Wild Type (WT)

NOTCH

Hedgehog

Smooth/Wingless

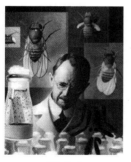

T.M. Hunt
(Courtesy of the Caltech Archives.)

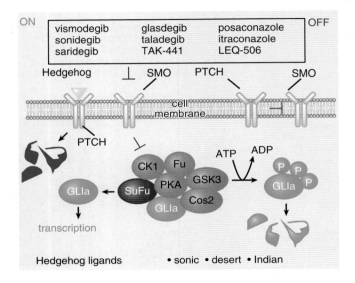

PHYSIOLOGY
- Canonical hedgehog (Hh) signaling occurs mostly in primary cilia (PC), which are immotile but are sensors for mechanical forces, chemicals, light, osmolarity, temperature, gravity.
- Inactive or poorly active in adults except during wound healing, other tissue repair
- Mediates progenitor/stem cell renewal
- Inappropriately activated in basal cell, brain, gastrointestinal, lung, breast, prostate cancer, one-third of malignant tumors
- Activation boosts antiapoptotic genes, angiogenic factors (angiopoietin-1,2), metastatic genes, cyclins D1,B1
- Suppresses apoptotic, cell adhesion, tight junction molecules
- Aberrant activation because of mutations in pathway components or sustained autocrine, paracrine activation
- Paracrine Hh signaling promotes tumorigenesis.
- Sensitive to environmental toxins, for example, piperonyl butoxide, which is common in household and agricultural pesticides

- The Hh pathway can be simplified into four fundamental components: (a) the ligand Hh, (b) the receptor Patched (Patch), (c) the signal transducer Smo, and (d) the effector transcription factor (Gli).
- Canonical Hh signaling occurs predominantly in the PC (Ng and Curran, 2011). PC are tubulin-polymerized immotile cilia that assemble from the centriole at the end of mitosis.
- Components of the Hh pathway concentrate in PC (Ramsbottom and Pownall, 2016; Roy, 2012), and a complex PC trafficking system regulates the interaction of Hh pathway components to enhance, or block, the Hh-initiated signal.

- **OFF State:** In the absence of Hh ligand, the receptor Patch prevents a GPCR-like protein—Smo—from entering the PC, repressing Smo activity.
- This allows the sequential phosphorylation of Gli by several kinases: protein kinase A (PKA), GSK3β, and CK1.
- Phosphorylated Gli is susceptible for ubiquitination by Skp-Cullin-F-box (SCF) protein/β-transducin repeat–containing protein (TrCP), which primes Gli to limited degradation in the proteasome.
- **ON State:** When Hh binds to Patch, it removes Patch from the PC, allowing Smo to enter the PC. The complex Hh–Patch is degraded in vesicles in the cytoplasm. The entry of Smo into the PC allows Smo activation.
- Active Smo abrogates phosphorylation and subsequent degradation of Gli. Full-length Gli translocates to the nucleus where it acts as a transcription factor for several target genes.
- Of note, Shh, Ihh, and Dhh ligands similarly activate the Hh pathway. Gli-1 does not undergo proteasomal degradation, and in the absence of ligand, Gli-2 is preferentially completely degraded in the proteasome, whereas Gli-3 is partially degraded, and hence Gli-1 and Gli-2 act mostly as transcription promoters and Gli-3 can act as a transcription repressor.
- Many human cancers, including brain, gastrointestinal, lung, breast, and prostate cancers, demonstrate inappropriate activation of this pathway.
- Paracrine Hh signaling from the tumor to the surrounding stroma has been shown to promote tumorigenesis.
- Targeted inhibition of Hh signaling may prove effective in the treatment and prevention of many types of human cancers.

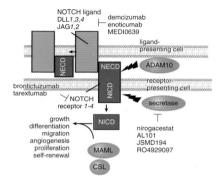

PHYSIOLOGY

- Essential for the development of nervous, cardiovascular, endocrine, respiratory system
- Signaling can be modified by glycosylation and fucosylation of NOTCH receptors, which can affect ligand–receptor interactions.
- Signaling also depends on endocytosis and trafficking of ligands and receptors, which can determine concentrations at cell surface.

CANCER-LINKED LESIONS IN NOTCH RECEPTORS

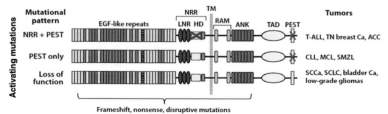

(Republished with permission of Annual Reviews, Inc., from Aster JC, Pear WS, Blacklow SC. The varied roles of Notch in cancer. *Annu Rev Pathol.* 2017 Jan 24;12:245-275.)

- NOTCH is a family of four transmembrane receptors (NOTCH 1–4) that are involved in cell–cell interaction and is found in most multicellular organisms.
- NOTCH signaling is critical to the differentiation and maintenance of several organs that include skin, blood, intestine, liver, and muscle.
- In cancers, mutations in NOTCH can be either activating or inactivating, resulting in oncogenic activity or loss of tumor suppressive function, respectively.
- The NOTCH receptor can be broadly structured into four regions: extracellular domain (NECD), transmembrane domain, intracellular domain (NICD), and the PEST domain located at the C-terminus.
- Two types of NOTCH ligands are known: Delta-like ligands (DLL1, DLL3, DLL4) and Jagged-like ligands (JAG1 and JAG2).
- The binding of the NOTCH ligand to its receptor results in a sequence of two proteolytic events. First, an ADAM family metalloprotease called ADAM10 cleaves the NOTCH protein just outside the plasma membrane. This releases the NECD that will continue to interact with the ligand.
- After the first cleavage, an enzyme called γ-secretase cleaves the remaining part of the NOTCH protein, releasing the NICD from the plasma membrane that translocates to the nucleus.
- In the nucleus, it interacts with DNA where it binds with transcription factors (RBP-J/CSL) and coactivators (Mastermind family, MamL) to induce transcription of target genes, promoting cell proliferation, differentiation, growth, migration, angiogenesis, and self-renewal.

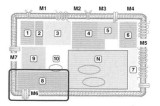

Caspases are activated by DRs and cellular "stress." They work through a network of intermediate molecules to cause cell death: Bid, BCL-2/BCL-Xl, ICAD, IAPS, Smac/Diablo, Omi/HtrA2, cytochrome c, Apaf1, AIF.

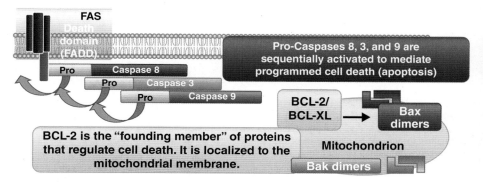

FAS

Death domain (FADD)

Pro Caspase 8

Pro Caspase 3

Pro Caspase 9

Pro-Caspases 8, 3, and 9 are sequentially activated to mediate programmed cell death (apoptosis)

BCL-2/ BCL-XL → **Bax dimers**

BCL-2 is the "founding member" of proteins that regulate cell death. It is localized to the mitochondrial membrane.

Mitochondrion

Bak dimers

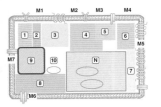

JAK-STAT inhibitors are used in the treatment of autoimmune diseases (rheumatoid arthritis and ulcerative colitis) as well as myeloproliferative disorders (polycythemia vera/essential thrombocytosis).

JAK/STAT has three main components:

1. Receptor is activated by cytokines or other chemical messengers.
2. JAKs (named because of its two nearly identical sequences) attached to the receptor bind phosphates and attract STAT proteins.
3. STATs form dimers and then translocate into nucleus where they bind to promoters, enhancers, and epigenetic regions to control transcription of target genes, microRNAs, and long noncoding RNAs.

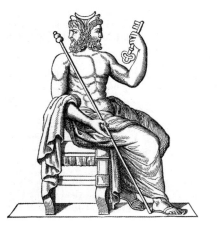

(From Alamy.)

- Among STAT target genes are those encoding SOCS (suppressor of cytokine signaling) factors, which inhibit JAK and contribute to termination of STAT signals.
- STATs can also induce apoptosis mainly by transcriptional activation of genes that encode proteins that trigger cell death process such as BCL-XL (B-cell lymphoma extra-large) and caspases (cysteine-dependent aspartate-directed proteases).
- Signaling through STAT factors in cancers can vary widely because of the many different STATs (e.g., STAT5 in hematologic cancers; STAT3 in breast cancer, head and neck cancer).
- STAT activity is also cross-regulated by protein kinases of MAPK, NF-κB, and PI3K pathways. Dysregulation of pathway may be caused by activating mutations in JAK or inactivation of SOCS.

PHYSIOLOGY
- JAK/STAT signaling mediated by JAK1–4 and STAT1–4,5A,5B,6
- STAT activity cross-regulated by MAPK, NF-κB, PI3K
- Essential in mammary gland, white blood, adipose, neuronal, cardiac, liver, stem cells
- Mediates nearly all immune regulatory processes.

NOTABLE BEHAVIORS IN CANCER
- Deregulation may be due to activating JAK mutations or inactivation of SOCS
- Deregulation may contribute to cancer, immune diseases
- Heterogeneous effects in cancer
- V617F in JAK2 seen in 50% to 95% of classical myeloproliferative neoplasms, polycythemia vera, essential thrombocytosis, primary myelofibrosis
- JAK/STAT activation in head and neck, high-grade ovarian epithelial cancers
- JAK2 amplification in gastric adenocarcinoma
- STAT1,2 drive antitumor immunity; STAT3 linked to cancer cell survival, immune suppression, and sustained inflammation in the tumor microenvironment

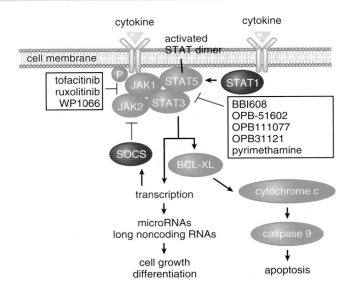

- JAK/STAT pathway transmits information through the cell membrane from chemical signals outside the cell and into genome DNA sites to regulate cell growth and differentiation.
- Many JAK/STAT pathways are important in white blood cells, mammary gland, adipocytes, neuronal cells, cardiomyocytes, hepatocytes, stem cells, and the like, and JAK/STAT deregulations may contribute to development of various diseases including immune diseases and cancers.
- There are four JAK family members (JAK1, JAK2, JAK3, and JAK4 or TYK2) and seven STAT family members (STAT1, STAT2, STAT3, STAT4, STAT5A, STAT5B, and STAT6).
- Receptor is activated by signal from cytokines (e.g., interferon, IL), growth factors, or other chemical messengers.
- After binding of ligand, cytokine receptors recruit JAKs, which phosphorylate each other and the receptor proteins, and create docking sites for STAT proteins, mostly STAT1, STAT3, and STAT5.
- STATs form dimers then translocate into nucleus. They then bind to different DNA sequence promoters, enhancers, and epigenetic regions to control transcription of target genes, microRNAs, and long noncoding RNAs and modify epigenetic markers and chromatin structures.

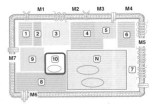

Three pathways promote Programmed Cell Death:

1. Extrinsic—TNF-Related Apoptosis-Inducing Ligand (TNF/TRAIL), FS7-associated surface antigen (FAS)
2. Intrinsic—Mitochondrial-based w/ DNA damage, ROS through BCL-2, BCL-XL, and dimers of Bax/Bak
3. CASPASE-independent pathway

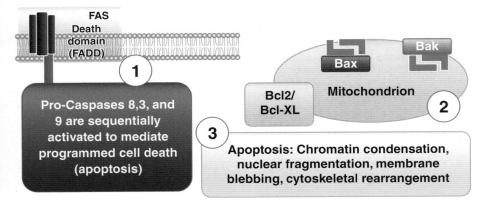

FAS
Death
domain
(FADD)

1 Pro-Caspases 8,3, and 9 are sequentially activated to mediate programmed cell death (apoptosis)

Bak

Bax

Mitochondrion

Bcl2/
Bcl-XL

2

3 Apoptosis: Chromatin condensation, nuclear fragmentation, membrane blebbing, cytoskeletal rearrangement

- DRs include Fas, TNFR, DR3, and DR4/5.
- After binding of ligands (e.g., FasL, TNF-α, AP0-3L/TWEAK, AP0-2L/TRAIL), DRs form dimers or trimers and recruit adaptor proteins that activate the caspase (casp) cascade via the mitochondria, which ultimately leads to apoptosis.
- Fas receptor (also known as apoptosis antigen 1: APO-1 or tumor necrosis factor receptor superfamily member 6 or TNFRSF6) forms the death-inducing signaling complex (DISC) as a result of ligand (FasL) binding.
- DISC is composed of the DR, adaptor protein FADD (Fas-associated protein with death domain), and caspase 8.
- TRAIL receptors 1 and 2 (TRAIL-R1 and -R2, also known as DR4 and DR5) are activated by TRAIL and also form DISC that leads to caspase cascade and apoptosis.
- DISC is inhibited by regulator FLIP (FLICE-like inhibitory protein, also known as caspase 8 and FADD-like apoptosis regulator or CFLAR).
- Other adaptor and regulator proteins mediate apoptotic signaling through different mechanisms, including RIP (receptor-interacting protein), DAXX (Fas death domain–associated xx), and ASK1 (apoptosis signal-regulating kinase 1, also known as MAP3K5).
- RIP activates BID (BH3 interacting-domain death agonist), a member of the proapoptotic BCL-2 (B-cell lymphoma 2) family.
- ASK1 is a member of the MAPKK kinase family and activates JNK (described in RAS pathway).
- Regulator proteins transport into the mitochondria and lead to a cascade of caspase activation that ultimately ends at apoptosis (PD).
- The process of apoptosis is regulated by several other signaling pathways:
  - AKT signaling through the inhibition of BAD
  - Abnormality sensor membrane detection system that responds to changes in pH or cellular damage and triggers cell death through BIM (BCL-2-like protein 11 proapoptotic regulator)
  - TP53 signaling through activation of BAX (BCL-2-like protein 4) proapoptotic regulator

- Proapoptotic factors act through metallothioneins (MTs), a family of proteins localized in the membrane of the Golgi apparatus that bind metals and control oxidative stress.
  - BCL-2 directly inhibits MT.
- In the absence of caspase activation, stimulation of DRs may lead to an alternative pathway of PD called necroptosis.
- Lenalidomide is a thalidomide analog and an FDA-approved inhibitor of TNF-α in multiple myeloma and mantle cell lymphoma.

NOTABLE BEHAVIORS IN CANCER
- Deregulated apoptosis linked to tumor initiation, progression, and chemoresistance
- Ligands of TNF receptors, that is, DRs, are considered as alternative to conventional chemo- or radiotherapy because of apoptotic effects independent of p53, which is often mutated in tumors.
- Some tumors are resistant to TRAIL-induced apoptosis, which is the most tumor cell–selective death mechanism.

PHYSIOLOGY
- Apoptosis is a key (silent/noninflammatory) mechanism maintaining tissue homeostasis.
- Apoptotic cells are swiftly cleared by phagocytosis to prevent release of intracellular components, which may inappropriately trigger signaling.
- DRs include Fas, TNFR, DR3, DR4/5.
- In the absence of caspase activation, DRs may trigger (inflammatory) necroptosis instead of apoptosis.

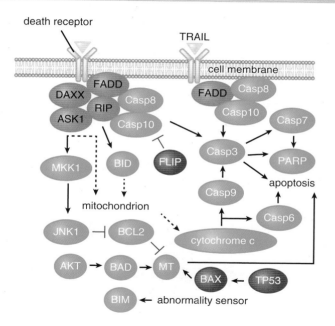

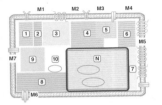

A remarkable number of factors are devoted to transcribing, controlling, and repairing DNA in order to maintain the integrity of the chromosomes, the cell cycle, and the thousands of "apps" present in every cell of the body.

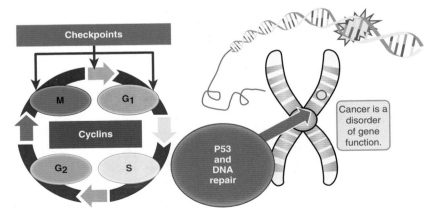

Checkpoints

M   G$_1$

Cyclins

G$_2$ S

P53 and DNA repair

Cancer is a disorder of gene function.

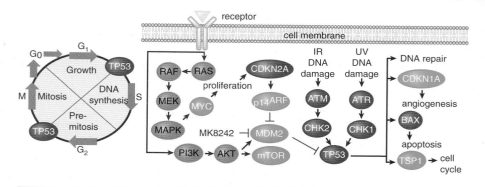

PHYSIOLOGY
- Cell cycle regulation mitigates genomic instability.
- TP53 regulates hundreds of genes and prevents genome damage.

NOTABLE BEHAVIORS IN CANCER
- Rare germline CHK2 mutations predispose to breast, colorectal cancer; somatic mutations seen in small subsets of malignancies.
- TP53 considered the most mutated genes in cancer; mutations can be inherited or somatic.
- TP53 may also be inactivated following loss of p14ARF, loss of upstream activators, loss of downstream effectors.

- *TP53* gene encodes for cellular tumor antigen (TA) or phosphoprotein p53 (name is in reference to apparent molecular mass of 53 kDa).
- Main function of TP53 is prevention of damage to genome, making it a tumor suppressor.
- TP53 acts as a transcriptional activator to several hundred genes.
- TP53 is an important regulator of G1/S and G2/M checkpoints.
- Considered the most frequently mutated gene in cancer
- Mutations may be inherited or sporadic.
- MDM2 is a negative regulator of TP53.
- MDM2 responsible for rapid turnover of TP53 (half-life 10–20 min)
  - MDM2 binds to TP53, blocking its transcriptional activity and initiating its transport out of the nucleus.
- MDM2 is activated by the PI3K pathway via AKT, but inhibited by RAS pathway via MYC and p14ARF.
- P14ARF is an ARF product of CDKN2A locus.
- MYC is a transcription factor that promotes proliferation by regulating the expression of specific target genes such as CDKN2A (cyclin-dependent kinase inhibitor 2A).
- Some tumors harbor amplifications of *MDM2* gene, which diminishes TP53 function.
- MDM2 inhibitors (e.g., MK-8242) are not effective against mutated TP53 because they function to silence normal TP53 function.
- Other mechanisms of TP53 inactivation include the following:
  - Loss of ARF (p14)
  - Loss of function of upstream activators including ATM and ATR, both activated by DNA double-strand breaks (DSBs)
  - Loss of function of downstream effectors, including angiogenesis regulator TSP1, apoptosis regulator BAX, and cell cycle regulator CDKN1A (cyclin-dependent kinase inhibitor 1A or p21)

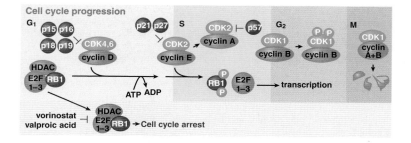

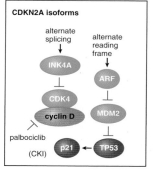

NOTABLE BEHAVIORS IN CANCER

- Loss of RB1 may result in deregulated cell proliferation.
- E2F overactivation may protect against effects of RB1 loss by inducing apoptosis.
- CDK mutation, hypermethylation, deletion are seen in various cancers.
- p15 is often deleted with p16, but may be crucial only in some leukemias.
- p57 inactivation is seen in some cancers.
- p21, p27 rarely mutated, but often downregulated; are good markers of progression and aggression.

- RB1 controls transition from G1 to S phase of cell cycle by binding to E2F1, E2F2, or E2F3 proteins and thereby repressing promoters of genes needed for the entrance into S phase.
- Phosphorylation performed by CDK4/cyclin D followed by CDK2/cyclin E is needed to inactivate RB1:
  - Activities of CDK4 and CDK2 protein kinases depend on the presence of their regulatory subunits, that is, cyclin D and cyclin E, respectively.
  - Regulatory activities of these subunits fluctuate in a coordinate fashion in the course of the cell cycle.
- Loss of RB1 function upsets cell cycle regulation and may lead to unrestrained cell proliferation.
- Overactivity of E2F factor may protect against loss of RB1 function by inducing apoptosis.
- RB1/E2F complex recruits histone deacetylase (HDAC) protein, which suppresses DNA synthesis.
- HDAC inhibitors valproic acid and vorinostat are FDA-approved neuroleptics currently in clinical trials for cancer.
- Two classes of protein inhibitors of CDKs also control cell cycle:
  - CIP/KIP comprises proteins p21 (*CDKN1A* gene), p27 (*CDKN1B* gene), and p57 (*CDKN1C* gene).
  - INK comprises proteins p15 (*CDKN2B* gene), p16 (*CDKN2A* gene), p18 (*CDKN2C* gene), and p19 (*CDKN2D* gene).
- In a wide range of human cancers, *CDKN2A* gene is inactivated by mutation, hypermethylation, or deletion (regarded as tumor suppressor gene).
- CDKN2B often deleted together with CDKN2A, which may only be crucial in certain leukemia types.
- Inactivation of CDKN1C may be relevant in a small range of cancers.

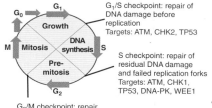

G₁/S checkpoint: repair of DNA damage before replication
Targets: ATM, CHK2, TP53

S checkpoint: repair of residual DNA damage and failed replication forks
Targets: ATM, CHK1, TP53, DNA-PK, WEE1

G₂/M checkpoint: repair of residual DNA damage before cell division
Targets: CHK1, MYT, WEE1

BRCA1,2

- Enable repair of DSBs

- Mutations in 5%–10% of all breast cancers; germline mutations in hereditary breast, ovarian cancer

- Indirectly targeted

- Therapeutic strategies quickly evolving with knowledge and understanding of DNA damage response (DDR)

DNA DAMAGE REPAIR PATHWAYS
(deficiencies drive carcinogenesis)

Damage	Damaging Agents	Repair Mechanism	Targets
Single-strand breaks	RTx Alkylating agents	Base excision	APE1 PARP
DSBs	RTx, Topo I inhibitors Nucleoside analog	Homologous recombination	ATR ATM
	RTx Topo I inhibitors	Nonhomologous end-joining	ATM DNA-PK
Bulky adducts	UV light Platinum agents	Nucleotide excision + translesion synthesis	ERCC1, XP polymerases
Substitutions insertions deletions	Replication errors Alkylating agents	Mismatch repair (MMR)	MLH, MSH MTH1, etc.

- Human cells are constantly exposed to exogenous and endogenous factors that might damage the genomic integrity and its correct transmission to the next generation.
- To respond to these threats, cells have developed an arsenal of enzymatic tools called DDR.
  - Modified bases and the DNA single-strand breaks (SSBs) are the most common form of DNA damage, and these are repaired by the base excision repair (BER) pathway.
  - For DNA DSBs, there are two major forms of repair: homologous recombination repair (HRR) and nonhomologous end-joining (NHEJ) pathways.
  - The nucleotide excision repair (NER) pathway deals with modified nucleotides that distort the structure of the double helix and it deals with UV-induced or platinum-induced DNA damage.
  - The MMR pathway deals with replication errors, including mismatch base-pairing as well as nucleotide insertions and deletions.
- DDR deficiency causes genetic aberrations that drive carcinogenesis.
- Breast cancer type 1 and type 2 (BRCA1 and BRCA2) are tumor suppressor genes that play an important role in the error-free repair of DNA DSBs, with BRCA1 also having a role in cell cycle checkpoint regulation.
- Cells with loss-of-function BRCA mutations have deficient HRR. Germline mutations in *BRCA1/2* genes are associated with hereditary breast and ovarian cancers. These mutations increase the risk of other cancers, including colon, pancreatic, and prostate. BRCA1/2 mutations account for 5% to 10% of all breast cancer cases.
- Cancer cells that have a reduced capacity to DNA repair pathway (that harbor a BRCA1 or BRCA2 mutation) are solely dependent on another, alternative pathway. This concept of synthetic lethality in cancer treatment is best demonstrated by sensitivity to poly (ADP-ribose) polymerase (PARP) inhibitors that are effective in patients with BRCA1/BRCA2-mutated cancers.

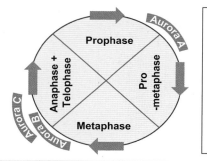

PHYSIOLOGY

- Regulates events in mitosis, including chromosome segregation, spindle checkpoint
- Aurora A required for centrosome function; expression regulated by p53; interacts with BRCA1
- Aurora B required for attachment of mitotic spindle to centromere; phosphorylates histone-H3; function regulated/modified by topoisomerase II, survivin, borealin, INCENP
- In mutually antagonistic relationship with TP53

NOTABLE BEHAVIORS IN CANCER

- Defects in chromosome segregation promote genetic instability, cell cycle progression, deregulated proliferation, tumorigenesis
- Mutated or amplified in cancer cells; diffusely distributed rather than concentrated at specific subcellular structures
- Overexpressed in cancer stem cells
- Stabilize MYC, reinforcing its tumorigenic properties
- Mutations in chromosome 20q13, which spans Aurora A, linked to poor prognosis
- Aurora A overexpression associated with poorer prognosis in specific cancers, predictive of distant metastasis in triple-negative breast cancer, others
- Aurora A variants Phe31/Ile and 91A-169G haplotype predict poor response to cisplatin-based therapy

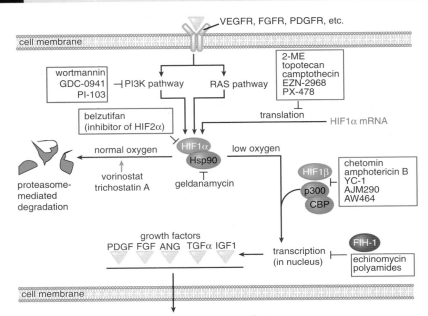

- Angiogenesis is a hallmark of cancer represented by the development of new blood vessels to keep up with the tumor needs, a process that is tightly controlled by pro- and antiangiogenic chemical signals.
- The **angiogenic switch** occurs when, in the hypoxic and inflammatory context of cancer, proangiogenic signals outweigh antiangiogenic signals, leading to tumor neovascularization. The shift in balance toward proangiogenic signals favors the abnormal and rapid growth and proliferation of local blood vessels.
- The sprouting of new blood vessels from the existing vasculature is the most widely investigated mode of new vessel formation in tumors. There are five other mechanisms of new vessel recruitment:
  ○ Vasculogenesis involves vessel formation by endothelial progenitor cells (EPCs), which are recruited from the bone marrow and/or are resident in vascular walls.
  ○ Intussusception is the splitting of preexisting vessels to give rise to daughter vessels.
  ○ Vessel co-option occurs when cancer cells grow around and co-opt the existing vasculature.
  ○ Vascular mimicry is a process in which cancer cells get incorporated into the blood vessel wall.
  ○ Tumor stem cell to EC differentiation occurs when cancer stem cell–like cells differentiate into ECs.
- Tumor angiogenesis, which allows for continued tumor growth, is often a deregulated process that results in incomplete, irregular, tortuous, and leaky capillaries. Tumor vessels exhibit bidirectional blood flow, are not constantly perfused, and tend to be larger than normal vessels with an altered surface area-to-volume ratio that results in poor nutrient delivery and waste removal.

Tumor hypoxia and inflammation trigger a proangiogenic switch that overcomes normal antiangiogenic mechanisms.

Angiogenic Switch

Activators, *e.g.*,	Inhibitors, *e.g.*,
HIF-1α	angiostatin
cytokines (IL-8)	tumstatin
growth factors	endostatin
inflammation	TSP-1
	TP53

(Modified from Hanahan D, Folkman J. Patterns and emerging mechanisms of the angiogenic switch during tumorigenesis. *Cell*. 1996;86:353–364. With permission from Elsevier.)

Angiogenic Effects Of Genetic Lesions

Gain of Function: Oncogenes		
PI3K	↑VEGF	↓TSP-1
HRAS	↑VEGF	
EGFR	↑VEGF, ↑FGF, ↑IL-8	
ERBB2	↑VEGF	
BCL2	↑VEGF	
SRC	↑VEGF	↓TSP-1
FOS	↑VEGF	
Loss of Function: Tumor Suppressors		
TP53	↑VEGF	↓TSP-1
VHL	↑VEGF	
PTEN	↑VEGF	
RB		↓TSP-1

Adapted from Wicki A, Christofori G. The angiogenic switch in tumorigenesis. In: Marmé D, Fusenig N, eds. *Tumor Angiogenesis: Basic Mechanisms and Cancer Therapy*. Springer; 2008:73.

NEW TUMOR VESSELS FORM BY

- Co-opting of existing vessels
- Differentiation of EPCs into new vessels
- Differentiation of cancer stem cell–like cells into ECs
- Incorporation of cancer cells into vessel walls
- Splitting of/sprouting from existing vessels

- Hypoxia or low oxygen tension results from uncontrolled proliferation of cancer cells in the absence of a functional and adequate vascular bed. It is a major driver of tumor angiogenesis.
  - The 2019 Nobel Prize was awarded to William Kaelin Jr., Sir Peter Ratcliffe, and Gregg Semenza for elucidating the importance of hypoxia-induced factors that respond to changes in oxygen levels.
  - Under normoxic conditions, hypoxia-inducible transcription factor-1 alpha (HIF-1α) subunits are subjected to von Hippel–Lindau (VHL)-directed protein degradation. VHL itself is a tumor suppressor, and VHL mutations have been implicated in malignancies such as renal cell carcinoma.
- Hypoxic conditions stabilize HIF-1α, allowing it to translocate to the nucleus and, along with HIF-1β, initiate the transcription of proangiogenic genes such as VEGF. Examples of proangiogenic signals secreted by tumors include the following:
  - Growth factors such as FGF, ANG, PDGF, VEGF
  - Cytokines such as IL-8
- TP53 negatively regulates angiogenesis by downregulating VEGF and other proangiogenic factors while increasing the expression of antiangiogenic signals such as thrombospondin 1 (TSP1). Loss of P53 function promotes VEGF expression and tumor angiogenesis, although the underlying mechanisms remain unclear and controversial.
- Other examples of endogenous inhibitors of angiogenesis include angiostatin, endostatin, tumstatin, and camstatin.

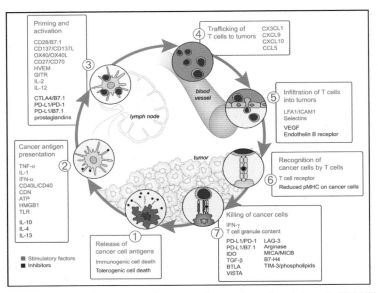

(Reprinted from Chen DS, Mellman I. Oncology meets immunology: the cancer-immunity cycle. *Immunity*. 2013;39(1):1–10. With permission from Elsevier.)

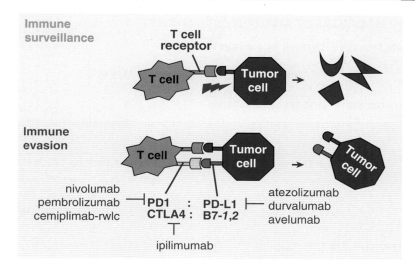

Immune surveillance

T cell receptor

T cell — Tumor cell →

Immune evasion

T cell — Tumor cell → Tumor cell

nivolumab
pembrolizumab
cemiplimab-rwlc ⊣ **PD1** : **PD-L1** ⊢ atezolizumab
CTLA4 : **B7-1,2** durvalumab
avelumab

⊤

ipilimumab

OTHER MODIFIERS OF ANTITUMOR IMMUNITY

Activating receptors (targeted by activators)
- 41BB
- CD28
- GITR
- OX40
- CD27
- HVEM

Inhibitory receptors (targeted by inhibitors)
- VISTA
- TIM-3
- BTLA
- LAG-3

Adoptive Cell Therapy	Chimeric Antigen Receptor T Cells (CAR-T)
Isolation of tumor-infiltrating lymphocytes (TILs)	Isolation of native T cells from patient
↓	↓
Expansion in vitro	Genetic engineering to express CAR
↓	↓
Reinfusion after lymphodepletion	Expansion in vitro
	↓
	Reinfusion

PD-1/PD-L1
- PD-1 is a cell surface protein involved in downregulating T-cell response, preventing autoimmunity under normal conditions.
- PD-1 is typically expressed on T cells and has two ligands, PD-L1 and PD-L2. Interactions between PD-1 and PD-L1 result in T-cell downregulation, impairment, exhaustion, and apoptosis, all of which lead to immune evasion. By hyperexpressing PD-L1, certain cancers can thwart the host immune system.

CTLA-4
- Cytotoxic T-lymphocyte antigen 4 (CTLA-4) is a receptor found exclusively on T cells. Activation of CTLA-4 downregulates T-cell activation and therefore immune response.
- CD80 (B7-1) and CD86 (B7-2) are ligands for CTLA-4, which when bound to each other prevent T-cell activation and immune signaling. Antibodies inhibiting CTLA-4, therefore, promote activation of effector T cells and downregulation of T regulatory cells (Tregs).
- When compared with PD1/PD-L1 blockade, CTLA-4 inhibition generally creates more immune-related toxicities. Where PD1/PD-L1–directed therapies depend on interaction of tumor and T cells, blocking CTLA-4 upregulates the earlier stages of T-cell activation and is independent of tumor interaction.

GITR
- Glucocorticoid-induced TNF receptor (GITR) is a receptor that belongs to the TNF receptor family, like OX-40 and 4-1BB. It is a costimulatory receptor that is highly expressed on Tregs, but is also found on T-effector cells, NK cells, macrophages, and dendritic cells. The ligand for GITR (GITRL) is expressed on antigen-presenting cells.

Immunotherapy *(continued)*

- Modulation of the GITR and GITRL results in intratumoral Treg inhibition and expansion of cytotoxic and memory CD8+ T cells.
- Antibodies to GITR or GITRL fusion proteins are in the early clinical phases of development and are being evaluated in solid tumors.
- Current clinical trials are evaluating GITR/GITRL modulation in combination with PD-1 or CTLA-4 inhibitors.

4-1BB

- 4-1BB (CD137) is a receptor that belongs to the TNF receptor family, like OX-40 and GITR. It is expressed on multiple immune cells with its downstream effect being activating and upregulating cytotoxic T cells. There is some evidence to suggest that activation of 4-1BB enhances antibody-dependent cell-mediated cytotoxicity (ADCC).
- There are currently two 4-1BB monoclonal antibodies being investigated—urelumab, a fully humanized immunoglobulin G (IgG)4, and utomilumab, a fully humanized IgG2—both of which are being investigated in clinical trials as a single agent and in combination with other immune checkpoint inhibitors.
- Although 4-1BB targeted therapies have a high potential for antitumor effect, there have been severe adverse immune-related events including hematologic toxicity and hepatitis.

OX40

- OX40 (CD134) is a costimulatory receptor that belongs to the TNF receptor family, like 4-1BB and GITR. It is expressed on T cells following their activation and promotes their survival during immune response.

- Modulation of OX40 or its ligand (OX40L) results in expansion and promotion of cytotoxic CD8+ T cells alongside nonregulatory CD4+ T cells.
- Several clinical trials with OX40 agonists are in clinical trials mostly in combination with PD1/PD-L1 and CTLA-4 inhibitors.

LAG3

- Lymphocyte activation gene 3 (*LAG-3*) (CD223) is a surface protein expressed on activated T cells, B cells, NK cells, and dendritic cells. LAG-3 is similar in structure to CD4 and binds to MHC Class II.
- LAG-3 functions as an immune checkpoint, and its interaction with MHC Class II inhibits downstream effects on CD4+ T cells. Increased LAG-3 expression on tumor samples has been identified in colorectal cancer and melanoma. By increasing LAG-3 expression, cancer cells can evade immune recognition and destruction.
- Blockade of LAG-3 leads to activation of T cells and inhibition of Tregs and upregulation of T-cell proliferation.
- LAG-3 antibodies are being investigated alone and in combination with PD-1 inhibitors.

TIM-3

- T-cell immunoglobulin mucin-3 (TIM-3) is a receptor expressed on a variety of cells including T cells, Tregs, NK cells, and dendritic cells. TIM-3+ T cells are considered dysfunctional and exhausted.
- TIM-3 functions as an immune checkpoint similar to, and possibly in conjunction with, PD-1.
- Patients previously failing PD-1 inhibitors have developed immune escape by upregulating TIM-3 as a response.

TIGIT

- T-cell immunoreceptor with Ig and ITIM domains (TIGIT) interacts with CD155 to suppress T cells and NKs, thereby inhibiting immune reactions, for example, antitumor immunity.
- Overexpressed on TA-specific CD8+ T cells and CD8+ TILs from patients with melanoma, breast cancer, non–small-cell lung carcinoma, colon adenocarcinoma, gastric cancer, acute myeloid leukemia, and multiple myeloma
- Dual blockade of TIGIT and PD-1 leads to increased cell proliferation, cytokine production, and degranulation of TA-specific CD8+ T cells and TIL CD8+ T cells.

ADOPTIVE CELL THERAPY

- Cell therapy involves the infusion of autologous or allogeneic immune cells used to target cancer cells.
- TILs were first used in the treatment of melanoma. TILs are essentially host immune cells that are isolated from the patient's own tumor sample. The TILs are expanded in vitro to a prespecified cell count and infused into the same patient after having received lympho-depleting chemotherapy. Patients have attained sustained complete response using TILs, and trials are ongoing.
- CAR-T use genetically altered autologous T cells that target certain antigens. The patient's native T cells are obtained peripherally through lymphopheresis. They are then genetically altered using a variety of different techniques to express a CAR. Once the CAR-T is generated, it is expanded in vitro and eventually infused back into a patient that has received lympho-depleting chemotherapy.
- CAR-T can target a variety of antigens, but the most common in development has been the B-cell antigen CD19.
- The use of CAR-T is being investigated in solid tumors with targets including EGFR, HER2, CEA, MSLN, PSMA, and CA125.

THYROID FUNCTION

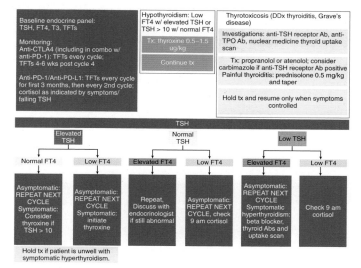

Baseline endocrine panel: TSH, FT4, T3, TFTs

Monitoring:
Anti-CTLA4 (including in combo w/ anti-PD-1): TFTs every cycle; TFTs 4-6 wks post cycle 4

Anti-PD-1/Anti-PD-L1: TFTs every cycle for first 3 months, then every 2nd cycle; cortisol as indicated by symptoms/ falling TSH

Hypothyroidism: Low FT4 w/ elevated TSH or TSH > 10 w/ normal FT4

Tx: thyroxine 0.5–1.5 ug/kg

Continue tx

Thyrotoxicosis (DDx thyroiditis, Grave's disease)

Investigations: anti-TSH receptor Ab, anti-TPO Ab, nuclear medicine thyroid uptake scan

Tx: propranolol or atenolol; consider carbimazole if anti-TSH receptor Ab positive
Painful thyroiditis: prednisolone 0.5 mg/kg and taper

Hold tx and resume only when symptoms controlled

TSH

Elevated TSH

- Normal FT4
  - Asymptomatic: REPEAT NEXT CYCLE
  - Symptomatic: Consider thyroxine if TSH > 10
- Low FT4
  - Asymptomatic: REPEAT NEXT CYCLE
  - Symptomatic: initiate thyroxine

Normal TSH

- Elevated FT4
  - Repeat, Discuss with endocrinologist if still abnormal
- Low FT4
  - Asymptomatic: REPEAT NEXT CYCLE, check 9 am cortisol

Low TSH

- Elevated FT4
  - Asymptomatic: REPEAT NEXT CYCLE
  - Symptomatic hyperthyroidism: beta blocker, thyroid Abs and uptake scan
- Low FT4
  - Check 9 am cortisol

Hold tx if patient is unwell with symptomatic hyperthyroidism.

(Data from Haanen J, Carbonnel F, Robert C, et al. Management of toxicities from immunotherapy: ESMO Clinical Practice Guidelines for diagnosis, treatment and follow-up. *Ann Oncol*. 2017;28:iv119–iv142.)

Management of Immune-Related Adverse Events (irAEs) (continued)

DIARRHEA AND COLITIS

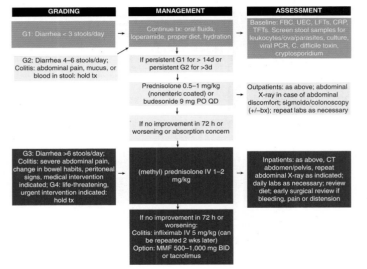

GRADING	MANAGEMENT	ASSESSMENT
G1: Diarrhea < 3 stools/day	Continue tx: oral fluids, loperamide, proper diet, hydration	Baseline: FBC, UEC, LFTs, CRP, TFTs. Screen stool samples for leukocytes/ova/parasites, culture, viral PCR, C. difficile toxin, cryptosporidium
G2: Diarrhea 4–6 stools/day; Colitis: abdominal pain, mucus, or blood in stool: hold tx	If persistent G1 for > 14d or persistent G2 for >3d ↓ Prednisolone 0.5–1 mg/kg (nonenteric coated) or budesonide 9 mg PO QD ↓ If no improvement in 72 h or worsening or absorption concern	Outpatients: as above; abdominal X-ray in case of abdominal discomfort; sigmoido/colonoscopy (+/–bx); repeat labs as necessary
G3: Diarrhea >6 stools/day; Colitis: severe abdominal pain, change in bowel habits, peritoneal signs, medical intervention indicated; G4: life-threatening, urgent intervention indicated: hold tx	(methyl) prednisolone IV 1–2 mg/kg ↓ If no improvement in 72 h or worsening: Colitis: infliximab IV 5 mg/kg (can be repeated 2 wks later) Option: MMF 500–1,000 mg BID or tacrolimus	Inpatients: as above, CT abdomen/pelvis, repeat abdominal X-ray as indicated; daily labs as necessary; review diet; early surgical review if bleeding, pain or distension

(Data from Haanen J, Carbonnel F, Robert C, et al. Management of toxicities from immunotherapy: ESMO Clinical Practice Guidelines for diagnosis, treatment and follow-up. *Ann Oncol.* 2017;28:iv119–iv142.)

HEPATITIS

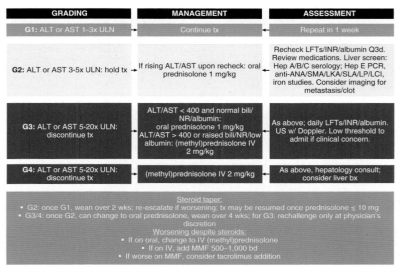

GRADING	MANAGEMENT	ASSESSMENT
G1: ALT or AST 1–3x ULN	Continue tx	Repeat in 1 week
G2: ALT or AST 3-5x ULN: hold tx	If rising ALT/AST upon recheck: oral prednisolone 1 mg/kg	Recheck LFTs/INR/albumin Q3d. Review medications. Liver screen: Hep A/B/C serology; Hep E PCR, anti-ANA/SMA/LKA/SLA/LP/LCI, iron studies. Consider imaging for metastasis/clot
G3: ALT or AST 5-20x ULN: discontinue tx	ALT/AST < 400 and normal bili/NR/albumin: oral prednisolone 1 mg/kg ALT/AST > 400 or raised bili/NR/low albumin: (methyl)prednisolone IV 2 mg/kg	As above; daily LFTs/INR/albumin. US w/ Doppler. Low threshold to admit if clinical concern.
G4: ALT or AST 5-20x ULN: discontinue tx	(methyl)prednisolone IV 2 mg/kg	As above, hepatology consult; consider liver bx

Steroid taper:
- G2: once G1, wean over 2 wks; re-escalate if worsening; tx may be resumed once prednisolone ≤ 10 mg
- G3/4: once G2, can change to oral prednisolone, wean over 4 wks; for G3: rechallenge only at physician's discretion

Worsening despite steroids:
- If on oral, change to IV (methyl)prednisolone
- If on IV, add MMF 500–1,000 bd
- If worse on MMF, consider tacrolimus addition

(Data from Haanen J, Carbonnel F, Robert C, et al. Management of toxicities from immunotherapy: ESMO Clinical Practice Guidelines for diagnosis, treatment and follow-up. *Ann Oncol.* 2017;28:iv119–iv142.)

Management of Immune-Related Adverse Events (irAEs) *(continued)*

PERIPHERAL NEUROLOGIC TOXICITY

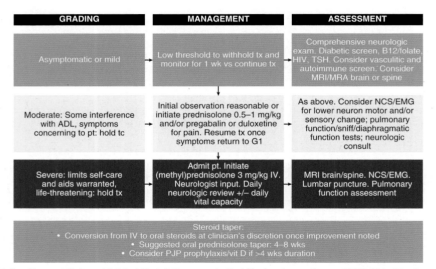

GRADING	MANAGEMENT	ASSESSMENT
Asymptomatic or mild	Low threshold to withhold tx and monitor for 1 wk vs continue tx	Comprehensive neurologic exam. Diabetic screen, B12/folate, HIV, TSH. Consider vasculitic and autoimmune screen. Consider MRI/MRA brain or spine
Moderate: Some interference with ADL, symptoms concerning to pt: hold tc	Initial observation reasonable or initiate prednisolone 0.5–1 mg/kg and/or pregabalin or duloxetine for pain. Resume tx once symptoms return to G1	As above. Consider NCS/EMG for lower neuron motor and/or sensory change; pulmonary function/sniff/diaphragmatic function tests; neurologic consult
Severe: limits self-care and aids warranted, life-threatening: hold tx	Admit pt. Initiate (methyl)prednisolone 3 mg/kg IV. Neurologist input. Daily neurologic review +/− daily vital capacity	MRI brain/spine. NCS/EMG. Lumbar puncture. Pulmonary function assessment

Steroid taper:
- Conversion from IV to oral steroids at clinician's discretion once improvement noted
- Suggested oral prednisolone taper: 4–8 wks
- Consider PJP prophylaxis/vit D if >4 wks duration

(Data from Haanen J, Carbonnel F, Robert C, et al. Management of toxicities from immunotherapy: ESMO Clinical Practice Guidelines for diagnosis, treatment and follow-up. *Ann Oncol.* 2017;28:iv119–iv142.)

PNEUMONITIS

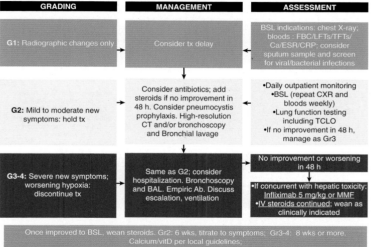

GRADING	MANAGEMENT	ASSESSMENT
G1: Radiographic changes only	Consider tx delay	BSL indications: chest X-ray; bloods : FBC/LFTs/TFTs/Ca/ESR/CRP; consider sputum sample and screen for viral/bacterial infections
G2: Mild to moderate new symptoms: hold tx	Consider antibiotics; add steroids if no improvement in 48 h. Consider pneumocystis prophylaxis. High-resolution CT and/or bronchoscopy and Bronchial lavage	•Daily outpatient monitoring •BSL (repeat CXR and bloods weekly) •Lung function testing including TCLO •If no improvement in 48 h, manage as Gr3
G3-4: Severe new symptoms; worsening hypoxia: discontinue tx	Same as G2; consider hospitalization. Bronchoscopy and BAL. Empiric Ab. Discuss escalation, ventilation	No improvement or worsening in 48 h → •If concurrent with hepatic toxicity: Infliximab 5 mg/kg or MMF •IV steroids continued; wean as clinically indicated

Once improved to BSL, wean steroids. Gr2: 6 wks, titrate to symptoms; Gr3-4: 8 wks or more. Calcium/vitD per local guidelines; pneumocystic prophylaxis: cotrimoxazole or inhaled pentamidine

(Data from Haanen J, Carbonnel F, Robert C, et al. Management of toxicities from immunotherapy: ESMO Clinical Practice Guidelines for diagnosis, treatment and follow-up. *Ann Oncol*. 2017;28:iv119–iv142.)

NEPHRITIS

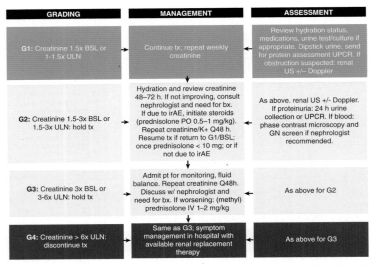

GRADING	MANAGEMENT	ASSESSMENT
G1: Creatinine 1.5x BSL or 1-1.5x ULN	Continue tx; repeat weekly creatinine	Review hydration status, medications, urine test/culture if appropriate. Dipstick urine, send for protein assessment UPCR. If obstruction suspected: renal US +/– Doppler
G2: Creatinine 1.5-3x BSL or 1.5-3x ULN: hold tx	Hydration and review creatinine 48–72 h. If not improving, consult nephrologist and need for bx. If due to irAE, initiate steroids (prednisolone PO 0.5–1 mg/kg). Repeat creatinine/K+ Q48 h. Resume tx if return to G1/BSL; once prednisolone < 10 mg; or if not due to irAE	As above. renal US +/- Doppler. If proteinuria: 24 h urine collection or UPCR. If blood: phase contrast microscopy and GN screen if nephrologist recommended.
G3: Creatinine 3x BSL or 3-6x ULN: hold tx	Admit pt for monitoring, fluid balance. Repeat creatinine Q48h. Discuss w/ nephrologist and need for bx. If worsening: (methyl) prednisolone IV 1–2 mg/kg	As above for G2
G4: Creatinine > 6x ULN: discontinue tx	Same as G3; symptom management in hospital with available renal replacement therapy	As above for G3

(Data from Haanen J, Carbonnel F, Robert C, et al. Management of toxicities from immunotherapy: ESMO Clinical Practice Guidelines for diagnosis, treatment and follow-up. *Ann Oncol.* 2017;28:iv119–iv142.)

SKIN RASH/TOXICITY

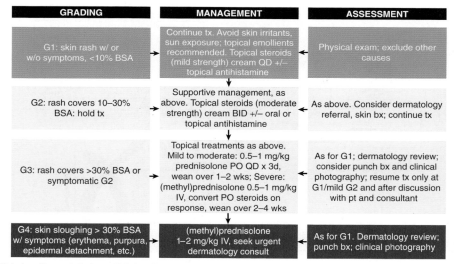

GRADING	MANAGEMENT	ASSESSMENT
G1: skin rash w/ or w/o symptoms, <10% BSA	Continue tx. Avoid skin irritants, sun exposure; topical emollients recommended. Topical steroids (mild strength) cream QD +/– topical antihistamine	Physical exam; exclude other causes
G2: rash covers 10–30% BSA: hold tx	Supportive management, as above. Topical steroids (moderate strength) cream BID +/– oral or topical antihistamine	As above. Consider dermatology referral, skin bx; continue tx
G3: rash covers >30% BSA or symptomatic G2	Topical treatments as above. Mild to moderate: 0.5–1 mg/kg prednisolone PO QD x 3d, wean over 1–2 wks; Severe: (methyl)prednisolone 0.5–1 mg/kg IV, convert PO steroids on response, wean over 2–4 wks	As for G1; dermatology review; consider punch bx and clinical photography; resume tx only at G1/mild G2 and after discussion with pt and consultant
G4: skin sloughing > 30% BSA w/ symptoms (erythema, purpura, epidermal detachment, etc.)	(methyl)prednisolone 1–2 mg/kg IV, seek urgent dermatology consult	As for G1. Dermatology review; punch bx; clinical photography

(Data from Haanen J, Carbonnel F, Robert C, et al. Management of toxicities from immunotherapy: ESMO Clinical Practice Guidelines for diagnosis, treatment and follow-up. *Ann Oncol.* 2017;28:iv119–iv142.)

HERITABLE GENOMIC CHANGES NOT CAUSED BY CHANGES IN DNA SEQUENCE

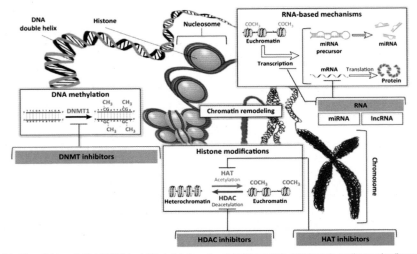

(Reprinted from Schiano C, Vietri MT, Grimaldi V, et al. Epigenetic-related therapeutic challenges in cardiovascular disease. *Trends Pharmacol Sci.* 2015;36:226–235. With permission from Elsevier.)

- **Epigenetics** are defined as heritable changes in the genome that are not caused by alterations in DNA sequence. The DNA exists in the form of chromatin, which is composed of units of nucleosomes. Nucleosome contains an octamer of histone core and the wrapping DNA of 147 bp.
- **Epigenetic mechanisms** include the DNA methylation, histone posttranslational modification, nucleosome restructure, and noncoding RNAs. These mechanisms regulate the switch between the active "euchromatic" and the suppressive "heterochromatic" transcription states.
  - **DNA methylation** involves the covalent transfer of a methyl group to the C-5 position of the cytosine ring of DNA by DNA methyltransferase (DNMT). In cancer cells, DNAs are globally hypomethylated but locally hypermethylated at the promoters of tumor suppressor genes. DNMT is overexpressed in many cancer types including leukemia and lung, breast, gastric, and colorectal cancers.
  - **DNMT inhibitors** azacitidine and decitabine are approved by the FDA for myelodysplastic syndrome. In clinical trials, low doses of DNMT inhibitors are used to sensitize cancer cells to radiation therapy, chemotherapy, and immunotherapies.
- **Histone modifications** are posttranscriptional modifications of the histones in a highly dynamic manner, mainly including histone acetylation, methylation, phosphorylation, ubiquitylation, and sumoylation.
- **Histone modifiers** respond to the upstream signals, recognize and bind (readers) to specific histone regions, and catalytically modify (writers or erasers) histone residues. Many of these modifications are abnormally regulated in cancer.

- **Histone acetylation** occurs on lysine residues on the histone tail and is associated with transcription activation. It is catalyzed by competing enzymes such as histone lysine acetyltransferases (HATs) and HDACs.
- **HDAC inhibitors** induce reexpression of tumor suppressors such as p21, p53, and NF-κB. Vorinostat, belinostat, and romidepsin are FDA-approved HDAC inhibitors for T-cell lymphoma. Panobinostat is another FDA-approved HDAC inhibitor in treating multiple myeloma.
- **Bromodomain and extraterminal protein (BET)** is a subfamily of bromodomains, which are histone acetylation readers. BET is a key player in transcriptional elongation and cell cycle progression. **BET inhibitors** have shown antitumor effects in NUT-midline carcinoma and hematologic malignancies in clinical trials.
- **Histone methylation** occurs on arginine and lysine residues and may either activate or inactivate transcription.
  - **EZH2** is the catalytic subunit of PRC2 complex, which trimethylates H3K27. High activity of EZH2 results in alterations in cell self-renewal and differentiation, cell cycle progression, and DNA repair. **EZH2 inhibitors** show antitumor and synthetic lethal effects with deficiency of SWI/SNF chromatin remodeling complexes.
  - **PRMT5**, a histone methyltransferase, is overexpressed in AML, lymphomas, glioblastomas, and lung and ovarian cancers. **PRMT5 inhibitors** are being tested in treating non-Hodgkin lymphoma and other solid tumors in clinical trials.
  - **Histone lysine demethylase LSD1** demethylates H3K4 and H3K9. **LSD1 inhibitors** induce apoptosis and prodifferentiation in leukemia cells in preclinical studies and are being tested in clinical trials.
- **Chromatin remodeling** uses the energy from ATP hydrolysis to mobilize and exchange histones, and thus allows open chromatin for gene activation. It is regulated by families of SWI/SNF, ISWI, and NuRD/Mi-2/CHD. The components of SWI/SNF family are tumor suppressors, for example, SNF5 loss leads to the development of malignant rhabdoid tumors. SWI/SNF deficiency is combined with other antitumor agents to reach therapeutic synthetic lethality in clinical trials.

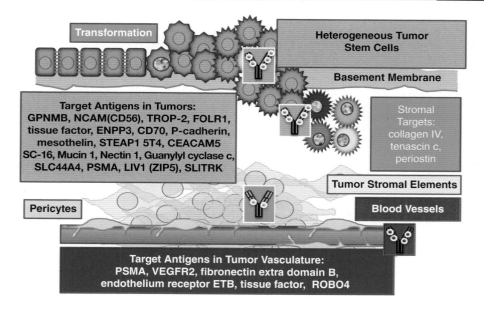

- Antibody–drug conjugates (ADCs) are a hybrid of cytotoxic drug and specific antibody joined by a linker.
- They provide targeted delivery of a cytotoxic agent with a reduced amount of toxicity.
- Their efficacy depends not on a mutation in the genome, but on a suitable marker on the cell surface.
- A successful ADC depends on a firmly attached cell surface antigen for the antibody to bind.
- These target antigens should be expressed at higher levels on tumor than on normal cells. Drug uptake should be via receptor-mediated endocytosis.
- Patients tend to benefit proportionally to the level of antigen expression on tumor cells.
- ADC specificity is limited because of the bystander effect, which causes cell death in adjacent cells that did not internalize the drug.
- Alternatively, ADCs can target the stroma and vasculature rather than the tumor itself.
- Commonly, the antibody portion is a human IgG1, which has the occasional benefit of activating antibody-dependent cellular cytotoxicity.
- The linker is a crucial piece of an ADC because it must not release the toxin in the bloodstream, while also releasing when necessary after endocytosis. The linker usually holds multiple molecules of a toxin to provide adequate cellular kill, with an optimal ratio of four toxin molecules to one antibody.
- Linker can be cleavable or noncleavable, with both approaches successfully used in drug development. (T-DM1 is a noncleavable linker.)
- The cytotoxic payload must be highly potent even at nanomolar concentrations, making traditional chemotherapy ineffective.
- Microtubule inhibitors such as auristatins cause G2/M-cell cycle arrest (brentuximab–vedotin).
- DNA-damaging agents such as calicheamicin work throughout the cell cycle (inotuzumab–ozogamicin).

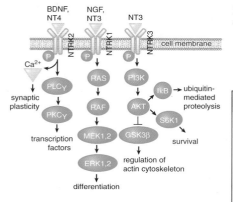

PHYSIOLOGY

- Neurotrophin receptors that regulate neuronal development and function; as well as memory, body weight, appetite, proprioception, pain, thermal regulation

NOTABLE BEHAVIORS IN CANCER

- Activation of downstream pathways drives tumor growth.
- Gene fusions pathognomonic in rare cancers such as congenital fibrosarcoma, secretory breast cancer, mammary analogue secretory carcinoma (MASC) of salivary gland
- Fusion partners include TPR, ETV6, TP53, TFG
- Mutations, splice variants, and overexpression also potentially tumorigenic
- Fusions also seen in papillary thyroid carcinoma (12%–14.5%), lung adenocarcinoma (3.3%), Spitzoid neoplasms (16%), pediatric high-grade glioma (40%)
- Highly responsive to first-generation inhibitors, but eventually acquire resistance, most commonly through solvent front mutations; resistance can be overcome by second-generation inhibitors currently in clinical trials; NGS needed to identify resistance mutations postprogression/nonresponse

- The tropomyosin-related kinases (TRKs) are neurotrophin receptors from the tyrosine kinase family and consist of three members: TRKA, TRKB, and TRKC, which are encoded by *NTRK1*, *NTRK2*, and *NTRK3* genes. The corresponding in vivo ligands are as follows: TRKA—neurotrophic growth factor (NGF) and neurotrophin-3 (NT-3); TRKB—brain-derived neurotrophic factor (BDNF) and neurotrophin-4 (NT-4); TRKC—NT-3 (Amatu et al., 2016).
- The TRK receptor family is involved in neuronal development, including the growth and function of neuronal synapses. In adults, TRK receptors regulate memory, body weight, appetite, proprioception, pain, and thermal regulation.
- Tropomyosin sequences cause activation of the kinase activity of the receptor with downstream activation of MAPK, PI3K, and PLCg pathways, resulting in cell proliferation, increased cell survival, and migration leading to tumor growth.
- Gene fusions involving the NTRK family are pathognomonic in rare cancers such as congenital fibrosarcoma, secretory breast cancer, and MASC of the salivary gland.
- *NTRK* gene fusions have been described across several cancer types with varying frequencies such as the following:
  - Papillary thyroid carcinoma (NTRK1—12%; NTRK3—14.5%)
  - Lung adenocarcinoma (3.3%)
  - Spitzoid neoplasms (16%)
  - Pediatric high-grade glioma (40%)

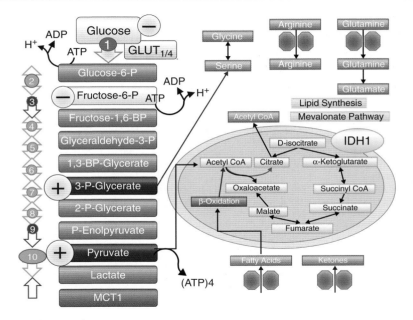

- Tumor cells metabolize glucose, lactate, pyruvate, hydroxybutyrate, acetate, glutamine, arginine, and fatty acids at much higher rates than nontumor tissue.
- These intermediary metabolites are released by catabolic cells, taken up by tumor cells, and used to replenish TCA-cycle intermediates and to fuel oxidative phosphorylation (reverse Warburg effect).
- Enasidenib (formerly AG-221) is a first-in-class inhibitor of mutated isocitrate dehydrogenase 2 (IDH2) and is now FDA-approved to treat acute myeloid leukemia.
- Similarly, ivosidenib, an inhibitor of IDH1, is FDA-approved in cholangiocarcinoma. The IDH enzyme normally metabolizes isocitrate into α-ketoglutarate. When mutated, it also converts α-ketoglutarate into 2-hydroxyglutarate, an oncometabolite that causes cell differentiation defects by impairing histone demethylation.
- Targeting glycolysis, mitochondrial metabolism, and amino acid metabolism with drug combinations holds promise as an antitumor strategy, and the following drugs are in early-phase trials:
  - Drugs inhibiting glycolysis—silibinin (GLUT1 inhibitor) (Ooi and Gomperts, 2015), TLN-232 (inhibits PKM2 dimerization and activity) (Vander Heiden et al., 2010)
  - Drugs inhibiting glutamine metabolism—CB-839 (Gross et al., 2014) and bis-2-(5-phenylacetamido-1,2,4-thiadiazol-2-yl)ethyl sulfide (BPTES) (Xiang et al., 2015) (glutaminase inhibitors)
  - Drugs targeting lactate, pyruvate, and acetyl-CoA production—AZD3965 (MCT1 inhibitor) (Polański et al., 2014)
  - Drugs degrading circulating arginine—ADI-PEG20 (Ascierto et al., 2005)

Targeted and Immunotherapy Agents

Color Key

Blue agents in late-stage clinical trial investigations (phases 2 and 3)

Green FDA-approved agents

Abbreviations

- ADC: antibody-drug conjugate
- 2HG: 2-hydroxyglutarate
- ADCC: antibody-dependent cell-mediated cytotoxicity
- AICARFT: aminoimidazole carboxamide ribonucleotide formyltransferase
- ALK: anaplastic lymphoma kinase
- ALT: alanine transaminase
- AML: acute myelogenous leukemia
- AST: aspartate aminotransferase
- BCRP: breast cancer resistance protein
- BRCA: BReast CAncer susceptibility gene
- CD: cytosine deaminase
- CPK: creatine phosphokinase
- CTLA4: cytotoxic T-lymphocyte–associated antigen 4
- DHFR: dihydrofolate reductase
- DVT: deep vein thrombosis
- EF: ejection fraction
- EGFR: epidermal growth factor receptor
- ERK2: extracellular signal–related kinase 2
- Fc: fragment crystallizable
- FGFR: fibroblast growth factor receptor
- FKBP-12: FK506-binding protein-12
- FLT3: FMS-related tyrosine kinase receptor-3
- FOLFIRI: folinic acid/fluorouracil/irinotecan
- GARFT: glycinamide ribonucleotide formyltransferase
- GE: gastroesophageal

- GERD: gastroesophageal reflux disease
- GGT: γ-glutamyl transferase
- GH: growth hormone
- GI: gastrointestinal
- GM-CSF: granulocyte-macrophage colony-stimulating factor
- GnRH: gonadotropin hormone-releasing hormone
- HCC: hepatocellular carcinoma
- HER2: human epidermal growth factor receptor 2
- IDH: isocitrate dehydrogenase
- Ig: immunoglobulin
- KDR: kinase insert domain receptor
- KRAS: Kirsten rat sarcoma
- LAR: low anterior resection
- LH: luteinizing hormone
- LVEF: left ventricular ejection fraction
- mAb: monoclonal antibody
- MAPK: mitogen-activated protein kinase
- mCRC: metastatic colorectal cancer
- MEK1: mitogen-activated protein kinase kinase 1
- MET: mesenchymal–epithelial transition
- MTC: medullary thyroid carcinoma
- mTOR: mammalian target of rapamycin
- NHL: non-Hodgkin lymphoma
- NSCLC: non–small-cell lung cancer
- NTRK: neurotrophic tropomyosin receptor kinase

- PARP: poly (ADP-ribose) polymerase
- PDGFR: platelet-derived growth factor receptor
- PD-L1: programmed death ligand 1
- PI3K: phosphatidylinositol 3-kinase
- pNET: pancreatic neuroendocrine tumor
- RAS: rat sarcoma virus
- RET: rearranged during transfection
- RTKs: receptor tyrosine kinases
- SCCHN: squamous cell carcinoma of the head and neck
- SCLC: small-cell lung cancer
- STS: soft-tissue sarcoma
- TCR: T-cell receptor
- TEN: toxic epidermal necrolysis
- TGF: transforming growth factor
- TRK: tropomyosin receptor kinase
- TS: thymidylate synthase
- VEGF: vascular endothelial growth factor
- VEGFR: vascular endothelial growth factor receptor
- VIP: vasoactive intestinal peptide

Adagrasib

- **Alias:** MRTX849
- **Type Mechanism:** Small-molecule inhibitor that targets the oncogenic KRAS substitution mutation, G12C, and covalently binds to cytosine 12 within the switch II pocket of GDP-bound KRAS G12C, resulting in inhibition of mutant KRAS-dependent signaling.
- **Drug Class:** KRAS inhibitor
- **Phase:** Phase 3
- **Indication:** Advanced colorectal cancer and NSCLC with KRAS G12C mutation
- **Dose:** RP2D: 600 mg po BID on empty stomach, 2 hours after previous meals or 1 hour prior to next meal
- **Metabolism:** Major CYP3A4 substrate; can also be potential inhibitor or P-gp, CYP2B6, 2C9, and 3A4.
- **Half-life:** ~23 hours
- **Side Effects:** Transaminitis with elevated ALT/AST, increased SCr, diarrhea, nausea/vomiting, fatigue
- **Clinical Pearls:** Possibly improved brain penetration by inhibition of P-gp-mediated drug efflux through blood–brain barrier

(Mok et al., 2021)

Afatinib Dimaleate

- **Brand Name:** Gilotrif
- **Type Mechanism:** A dimaleate salt form of afatinib, an orally bioavailable anilinoquinazoline derivative and inhibitor of the RTK EGFR (ErbB). Upon administration, afatinib selectively and irreversibly binds to and inhibits the epidermal growth factor receptors 1 (ErbB1; EGFR), 2 (ErbB2; HER2), and 4 (ErbB4; HER4), and certain EGFR mutants, including those caused by EGFR exon 19 deletion mutations or exon 21 (L858R) mutations. In addition, afatinib inhibits the EGFR T790M gatekeeper mutation, which is resistant to the treatment with the first-generation EGFR inhibitors. EGFR, HER2, and HER4 are RTKs that belong to the EGFR superfamily.
- **Drug Class:** EGFR inhibitor
- **Mechanism of Action:** A TKI that covalently binds to EGFR (ErbB1), HER2 (ErbB2), and HER4 (ErbB4) to irreversibly inhibit tyrosine kinase autophosphorylation and downregulate ErbB signaling
- **FDA Approval Date:** July 12, 2013
- **Indications:** Metastatic EGFR mutation–positive NSCLC and metastatic squamous cell lung cancer

- **Dose:** 40 mg PO daily. Administer ≥1 hour before or 2 hours after a meal.
- **Half-life:** 37 hours
- **Metabolism:** P-glycoprotein/ABCB1 major substrate
- **Side Effects:** Acneiform eruption, skin rash, paronychia, xeroderma, pruritis, cheilitis, diarrhea, stomatitis, nausea, vomiting, lymphocytopenia, transaminitis, hyperbilirubinemia, hypokalemia
- **Clinical Pearls:** Binding to T790M can lead to longer time to resistance.

Alectinib

- **Alias:** AF802; CH5424802; RG7853; RO5424802
- **Brand Name:** Alecensa
- **Type Mechanism:** A tyrosine kinase receptor inhibitor that inhibits ALK and RET, resulting in decreased tumor cell viability. Alectinib is more potent than crizotinib against ALK and can inhibit most of the clinically observed acquired ALK resistance mutations to crizotinib.
- **Drug Class:** Tyrosine kinase receptor inhibitor

- **Mechanism of Action:** ALK and RET inhibitors
- **FDA Approval Date:** December 11, 2015
- **Indications:** Metastatic NSCLC with ALK-positive mutation
- **Dose:** 600 mg BID with food
- **Half-life:** 33 hours ; M4-active metabolite 31 hours
- **Metabolism:** Minor CYP3A4 substrate
- **Side Effects:** Edema, bradycardia, fatigue, headache, rash, hyperglycemia, hypophosphatemia, transaminitis, hyperbilirubinemia, muscle pain, increased CPK, increased SCr, constipation
- **Clinical Pearls:** Dose adjustment needed for both grade 2 transaminitis and hyperbilirubinemia.

Apatinib

- **Alias:** YN968D1; rivoceranib (international nonproprietary name)
- **Type Mechanism:** Orally bioavailable VEGFR2 (KDR) inhibitor; also mildly inhibits RET, KIT, and SRC
- **Drug Class:** Antiangiogenic TKI
- **Mechanism of Action:** Selectively inhibits VEGFR2

- **Phase:** Phase 3 gastric cancer and HCC; FDA granted orphan status in adenoid cystic carcinoma; phase 2 in CRC
- **FDA Approval Date:** Orphan status for adenoid cystic carcinoma
- **Indications:** Gastric cancer, CRC, adenoid cystic carcinoma, HCC
- **Dose:** 850 mg daily in 2 divided doses; optimum dose seen is 500 mg daily.
- **Half-life:** 9 hours
- **Metabolism:** Extensively by CYP3A4/5
- **Side Effects:** HTN, hand-foot syndrome, diarrhea, anemia, thrombocytopenia, neutropenia, proteinuria, fatigue
- **Clinical Pearls:** UGT1A4 and UT2B7 deficiency may affect metabolism of apatinib.

(Du et al., 2020)

Atezolizumab

- **Alias:** MPDL3280A; RO5541267
- **Brand Name:** Tecentriq
- **Type Mechanism:** A humanized mAb inhibiting PD-L1
- **Drug Class:** A humanized mAb immune checkpoint inhibitor
- **Mechanism of Action:** Binds to PD-L1 to selectively prevent the interaction between the programmed cell death-1 (PD-1) and B7.1. PD-L1 is an immune checkpoint protein expressed on tumor cells and tumor-infiltrating cells and downregulates antitumor T-cell function by binding to PD-1 and B7.1; blocking PD-1 and B7.1 interactions restores antitumor T-cell function.
- **FDA Approval Date:** May 18, 2016
- **Indications:** PD-L1–positive triple-negative breast cancer (TNBC); urothelial cancer ineligible for platinum-containing chemotherapy; metastatic NSCLC; SCLC; metastatic HCC; metastatic melanoma
- **Dose:** 840 mg IV Q 2 weeks; 1,200 mg IV Q 3 weeks; or 1,680 mg IV Q 4 weeks
- **Half-life:** 27 days
- **Side Effects:** Peripheral edema, fatigue, skin rash, hyponatremia, decreased appetite, transaminitis, hyperbilirubinemia, infection
- **Clinical Pearls:** When combining with chemotherapy, administer atezolizumab first

Avelumab

- **Alias:** MSB0010718C
- **Brand Name:** Bavencio
- **Type Mechanism:** Fully human mAb that binds to PD-L1 to selectively prevent the interaction between PD-1 and 7.1 receptors,

resulting in the restoration of antitumor T-cell function
- **Drug Class:** Anti–PD-L1 mAb
- **FDA Approval Date:** March 23, 2017
- **Indications:** Metastatic Merkel cell carcinoma; locally, advanced, or metastatic urothelial carcinoma following platinum therapy; advanced renal cell carcinoma (RCC)
- **Dose:** 10 mg/kg IV over 60 minutes Q 2 weeks (for gestational trophoblastic neoplasia chemotherapy resistant) or 800 mg (FLAT dose) IV Q 2 weeks; should premedicate with acetaminophen and diphenhydramine for the first four infusions
- **Half-life:** 6.1 days
- **Side Effects:** Peripheral edema, HTN, fatigue, dizziness, skin rash, nausea, diarrhea, hyponatremia, decreased appetite, abdominal pain, transaminitis, arthralgia, infusion-related reaction with chills, fevers

Axitinib

- **Alias:** AG-013736
- **Brand Name:** Inlyta
- **Type Mechanism:** Selective second-generation, orally bioavailable inhibitor of VEGFRs (VEGFR-1, VEGFR-2, and VEGFR-3), PDGFR, and KIT
- **Drug Class:** VEGF TKI
- **FDA Approval Date:** January 27, 2012
- **Indications:** Advanced RCC; off-label use for differentiated thyroid cancer
- **Dose:** Optimum dose is 10 mg PO BID; recommend to dose escalate Q 2 weeks starting at 5 mg.
- **Half-life:** 2 to 6 hours
- **Metabolism:** Major CYP3A4 substrate and UGT1A1 substrate
- **Side Effects:** Diarrhea, HTN, fatigue, decreased appetite, palmar–plantar erythrodysesthesia, skin rash, stomatitis, hypothyroidism, transaminitis, increased SCr, nausea/vomiting
- **Clinical Pearls:** Dysphonia (hoarseness) may occur while taking. Advise patients to avoid irritants and to drink plenty of fluids.

Bemarituzumab

- **Alias:** FPA144
- **Type Mechanism:** A glycoengineered, humanized mAb directed against the FGFR2b that specifically binds to and inhibits FGFR2b on tumor cell surfaces, which prevents FGFR2 from binding to its ligands, FGFR2b activation, and

the activation of FGFR2b-mediated signal transduction pathways. The binding of bemarituzumab to FGFR2b protein also induces ADCC against FGFR2b-expressing tumor cells.

- **Phase:** Phase 2/3
- **Indications:** GE adenocarcinoma or gastric carcinoma with FGFR2b overexpression
- **Dose:** 15 mg/kg IV Q 2 weeks in combination with mFOLFOX
- **Half-life:** 12.8 days
- **Side Effects:** Fatigue, nausea, dry eyes, anemia, neutropenia, increased AST, vomiting, infusion reaction

(Catenacci et al., 2020)

Bevacizumab

- **Brand Name:** Avastin
- **Type Mechanism:** A recombinant humanized mAb directed against the VEGF, a proangiogenic cytokine
  - Binds to VEGF and inhibits receptor binding, thereby preventing the growth and maintenance of tumor blood vessels
- **Drug Class:** VEGF inhibitor
- **FDA Approval Date:** February 26, 2004
- **Indications:** Colon, lung, and renal carcinomas and glioblastoma multiforme
- **Dose:** 5 to 10 mg/kg IV Q 2 weeks or 15 mg/kg IV Q 3 weeks
- **Half-life:** 20 days
- **Side Effects:** HTN, severe or fatal hemorrhage (GI bleed, hemoptysis, central nervous system [CNS] bleed), bowel perforation, fistulas/abscess formation, proteinuria
- **Clinical Pearls:** Have patients monitor blood pressure and bring the log to appointments. Avoid use in patients with severe hypertension requiring multiple antihypertensive medications for control.

Binimetinib

- **Alias:** ARRY-162; MEK162; ARRY-43162
- **Type Mechanism:** An orally available inhibitor of MEK1/2 prevents the activation of MEK1/2-dependent effector proteins and transcription factors, which may result in the inhibition of growth factor–mediated cell signaling. This may eventually lead to an inhibition of tumor cell proliferation and an inhibition in the production of various inflammatory cytokines, including IL-1, IL-6, and tumor necrosis factor (TNF).
- **Drug Class:** MEK1/2 inhibitor

- **FDA Approval Date:** June 27, 2018
- **Indications:** Unresectable or metastatic melanoma; off-label use for metastatic, refractory, RAS WT, and BRAF V600E–mutant CRC
- **Dose:** 45 mg PO Q 12 hours
- **Half-life:** 3.5 hours
- **Metabolism:** BCRP/ABCG2 substrate; UGT1A1 substrate
- **Side Effects:** Skin rash, fatigue, dermatitis acneiform, peripheral edema, diarrhea, nausea, elevated CPK, anemia, increased GGT, transaminitis
- **Clinical Pearls:** Use in combination with encorafenib in melanoma.

Cabozantinib

- **Alias:** XL-184
- **Brand Name:** Cometriq (for MTC); Cabometyx (for HCC and RCC)
- **Type Mechanism:** Potent inhibitor of RTKs, including AXL, FLT-3, KIT, MET, RET, TIE-2, TRKB, and VEGFR-1, VEGFR-2, and VEGFR-3. It induces apoptosis of cancer cells and suppresses tumor growth, metastasis, and angiogenesis.
- **Drug Class:** Multikinase inhibitor
- **Mechanism of Action:** Multikinase inhibitor

- **FDA Approval Date:** November 29, 2012
- **Indications:** Advanced HCC and RCC; metastatic MTC
- **Dose:** HCC dosing: 60 mg PO daily; RCC dosing: 40 mg PO daily with nivolumab or 60 mg PO daily (monotherapy); MTC dosing: 140 mg PO daily
- **Half-life:** Cometriq = ~55 hours; Cabometyx = ~99 hours
- **Metabolism:** Major CYP3A4 substrate
- **Side Effects:** Hemorrhage, perforation/fistula (U.S. box warning), HTN, stomatitis, palmar–plantar erythrodysesthesia, decreased appetite, weight loss, nausea/vomiting, diarrhea, tiredness and weakness, change in hair color, liver dysfunction (hyperbilirubinemia, transaminitis, increases alkaline phosphatase)
- **Clinical Pearls:** May affect the rate of wound healing; patients should notify doctor before surgery or dental work; moderate-to-high emetogenicity.

Cetuximab

- **Alias:** C225; IMC-C225
- **Brand Name:** Erbitux
- **Type Mechanism:** A recombinant human/mouse chimeric mAb that binds specifically

to EGFR (HER1, c-ErbB-1) and competitively inhibits the binding of EGF and other ligands

- **Drug Class:** EGFR inhibitor
- **FDA Approval Date:** February 12, 2004
- **Indications:** KRAS WT CRC; SCCHN; off label for RAS WT, BRAF V600E–mutated CRC, SCC of the penis, and SCC of the skin
- **Dose:** Weekly dose: 400 mg/m^2 as 120-minute IV infusion as an initial dose, followed by 250 mg/m^2 infused over 30 minutes weekly. Biweekly dose: 500 mg/m^2 IV over 120 minutes once Q 2 weeks
- **Half-life:** ~112 hours
- **Side Effects:** Infusion reactions (U.S. box warning), nausea/vomiting, diarrhea, skin problems (acneiform rash, pruritus), hypomagnesemia, stomatitis, lung disease (dyspnea, cough), fatigue, neutropenia, transaminitis, palmar–plantar erythrodysesthesia, xeroderma
- **Clinical Pearls:** Severity of acneiform rash can be minimized with the use of topical steroid cream, topical antibiotic gel, and doxycycline.

Crizotinib

- **Brand Name:** Xalkori
- **Type Mechanism:** A tyrosine kinase receptor inhibitor that inhibits ALK, HGFR (c-MET), ROS1 (c-ros), and recepteur d'origine nantais (RON). It induces apoptosis and inhibits proliferation and ALK-mediated signaling in ALCL-derived cell lines.
- **FDA Approval Date:** August 26, 2011
- **Indications:** Locally advanced or metastatic ALK-positive NSCLC
- **Dose:** 250 mg PO BID
- **Half-life:** 42 hours
- **Metabolism:** Major CYP3A4 substrate and P-glycoprotein; moderate CYP3A4 inhibitor
- **Side Effects:** Edema, vision problems (diplopia, blurred vision), nausea/vomiting, diarrhea, dysphagia, GERD, reflux esophagitis, skin rash, swelling of hands or feet, fatigue, dizziness, transaminitis
- **Clinical Pearls:** Advise patients to exercise caution when driving or operating machinery because of the risk of developing visual changes such as floaters, blurred vision, light sensitivity, or flashes of light.

Dabrafenib

- **Alias:** GSK2118436
- **Brand Name:** Tafinlar
- **Type Mechanism:** Selectively binds to and inhibits the activity of B-raf, which may inhibit the proliferation of tumor cells that contain a mutated *BRAF* gene

- **FDA Approval Date:** March 29, 2013
- **Indications:** Melanoma with BRAF V600E or V600K; metastatic NSCLC with BRAF V600E; metastatic, anaplastic thyroid cancer with BRAF V600E in combination with trametinib
- **Dose:** 150 mg PO BID on fasting stomach at least 1 hour before or 2 hours after meals
- **Half-life:** Parent drug 8 hours; hydroxy-dabrafenib (active metabolite) 10 hours; desmethyl-dabrafenib (active metabolite) 21 to 22 hours
- **Metabolism:** Major CYP2C8 and CYP3A4 substrates; moderate CYP3A4 inducer
- **Side Effects:** Keratoacanthoma and SCC, fatigue, arthralgias, pyrexia, papilloma, hyperglycemia, hyperkeratosis, palmar–plantar erythrodysesthesia, skin rash, hypophosphatemia
- **Clinical Pearls:** Corticosteroids may be used as an effective fever prophylaxis when fever occurs.

Durvalumab

- **Alias:** MEDI4736
- **Brand Name:** Imfinzi
- **Type Mechanism:** A human IgG1κ mAb that blocks PD-L1 binding to PD-1 and CD80 (B7.1); PD-L1 blockade leads to increased T-cell activation, allowing T cells to kill tumor cells. PD-L1 is an immune checkpoint protein expressed on tumor cells and tumor-infiltrating cells and downregulates antitumor T-cell function by binding to PD-1 and B7.1; blocking PD-1 and B7.1 interactions restores antitumor T-cell function.
- **Drug Class:** Anti–PD-L1 mAb
- **FDA Approval Date:** May 1, 2017
- **Indications:** Unresectable NSCLC and extensive stage SCLC; locally advanced or metastatic urothelial carcinoma
- **Dose:** 10 mg/kg IV Q 2 weeks; may use flat dosing of 1,500 mg IV Q 3 to 4 weeks for patients ≥30 kg
- **Half-life:** ~18 days
- **Side Effects:** Fatigue, skin rash, muscle pain, peripheral edema, abdominal pain, lymphocytopenia, constipation, immune-mediated pneumonitis

Encorafenib

- **Alias:** LGX818
- **Brand Name:** Braftovi
- **Type Mechanism:** An ATP-competitive inhibitor of protein kinase B-raf (BRAF) that

suppresses the MAPK pathway and targets BRAF V600E, V600D, and V600K. It has a longer dissociation half-life than other BRAF inhibitors, allowing for sustained inhibition. BRAF V600 mutations result in constitutive activation of the BRAF pathway (which may stimulate tumor growth); BRAF inhibition inhibits tumor cell growth.

- **Drug Class:** BRAF inhibitor
- **FDA Approval Date:** April 8, 2020
- **Indications:** Metastatic, BRAF V600E–mutant CRC and unresectable/metastatic BRAF V600E– or V600K-mutated melanoma
- **Dose:** CRC: 300 mg PO daily with cetuximab; melanoma: 450 mg PO daily with binimetinib
- **Half-life:** 3.5 hours
- **Metabolism:** Major CYP3A4 substrate
- **Side Effects:** Anemia, hyperglycemia, fever, increased lipase, HTN, fatigue, nausea, arthralgia, palmar–plantar erythrodysesthesia, acneiform eruption, alopecia, hyperkeratosis, xeroderma, arthralgia, increased SCr

Entrectinib

- **Alias:** RXDX-101
- **Brand Name:** Rozlytrek

- **Type Mechanism:** Inhibits TRK receptors such as TRKA, TRKB, and TRKC. TRKA, TRKB, and TRKC are encoded by NTRK genes *NTRK1*, *NTRK2*, and *NTRK3*, respectively. It also inhibits proto-oncogenic tyrosine protein kinase ROS1 and ALK. M5 (the major active entrectinib metabolite) demonstrated similar activity (in vitro) against TRK, ROS1, and ALK. Fusion proteins that include TRK, ROS1, or ALK domains act as oncogenic drivers to promote hyperactivation of downstream signaling pathways, resulting in unchecked cell proliferation.
- **Drug Class:** TRK inhibitor
- **FDA Approval Date:** August 15, 2019
- **Indications:** Metastatic NSCLC with ROS1 positive; all metastatic, unresectable solid tumors with *NTRK* gene fusion
- **Dose:** 600 mg PO daily
- **Half-life:** Entrectinib = 20 hours
  - M5 active metabolite = 40 hours
- **Metabolism:** Major CYP3A4 substrate
- **Side Effects:** Edema, hypotension, fatigue, cognitive dysfunction, sleep disorder, myasthenia, hyperuricemia, dysgeusia, constipation, diarrhea, increased lipase, anemia, lymphocytopenia, neutropenia myalgia, arthralgia, visual disturbance, elevated SCr, cough, fever

- **Clinical Pearls:** Avoid grapefruit or grapefruit juice as it may increase the levels of entrectinib.

Erdafitinib

- **Alias:** JNJ-42756493
- **Brand Name:** Balversa
- **Type Mechanism:** A pan-FGFR kinase inhibitor that binds to and inhibits FGFR1, FGFR2, FGFR3, and FGFR4 enzyme activity. Erdafitinib also binds to RET, CSF1R, PDGFRα, PDGFRβ, FLT4, KIT, and VEGFR2. FGFR inhibition results in decreased FGFR-related signaling and decreased cell viability in cell lines expressing FGFR genetic alterations, including point mutations, amplifications, and fusions.
- **Drug Class:** FGFR inhibitor
- **FDA Approval Date:** April 14, 2019
- **Indications:** Advanced/metastatic urothelial carcinoma with susceptible FGFR genetic alteration
- **Dose:** 8 mg PO daily for 14 days; if serum phosphate $\leq$ 5.5 mg/dL, and no ocular toxicity $\geq$ grade 2 common terminology criteria for adverse events (CTCAEs), then increase dose 9 mg PO daily.
- **Half-life:** 59 hours
- **Metabolism:** Major CYP2C9 and CYP3A4 substrates

- **Side Effects:** Fatigue, onycholysis, xeroderma, alopecia, palmar–plantar erythrodysesthesia, paronychia, nail discoloration, hyperphosphatemia, hyponatremia, stomatitis, diarrhea, xerostomia, dysgeusia, anemia, thrombocytopenia, leukopenia, transaminitis, dry eyes syndrome, central serous retinopathy, blurred vision, elevated SCr, myalgia

Erlotinib

- **Alias:** OSI-774; CP 358774
- **Brand Name:** Tarceva
- **Type Mechanism:** Reversibly binds to the intracellular catalytic domain of EGFR and inhibits overall HER1/EGFR tyrosine kinase. Active competitive inhibition of ATP inhibits downstream signal transduction of ligand-dependent HER1/EGFR activation.
- **Drug Class:** EGFR inhibitor
- **FDA Approval Date:** November 18, 2004
- **Indications:** Metastatic NSCLC with EGFR exon 19 deletions or exon 21 substitution mutations; locally advanced, unresectable, or metastatic pancreatic cancer (in combination with gemcitabine); off-label use for advanced papillary RCC
- **Dose:** 150 mg once daily (NSCLC) and 100 mg once daily (pancreatic cancer) on empty stomach 1 hour before or 2 hours after meals

- **Half-life:** 36 hours
- **Metabolism:** Major CYP3A4 and CYP1A2 substrates
- **Side Effects:** Rash (acne vulgaris, pruritus), diarrhea, paronychia (hair and nail changes), fatigue, weakness, back pain, cough, dyspnea, conjunctivitis, chest pain, xeroderma, anorexia, nausea, mucositis, dry eyes syndrome, increased ALT and GGT
- **Clinical Pearls:** Severity of acne-form rash can be minimized with the use of topical steroid cream, topical antibiotic gel, and doxycycline; encourage smoking cessation before start because smoking can make the drug less effective.

Everolimus

- **Alias:** RAD001
- **Brand Name:** Afinitor
- **Type Mechanism:** An mTOR inhibitor that has antiproliferative and antiangiogenic properties. Reduces protein synthesis and cell proliferation by binding to the FKBP-12, an intracellular protein, to form a complex that inhibits activation of mTOR serine-threonine kinase activity. Also reduces angiogenesis by inhibiting VEGF and hypoxia-inducible factor (HIF-1) expression.

- **Drug Class:** mTOR inhibitor
- **FDA Approval Date:** March 30, 2009
- **Indications:** Advanced RCC, neuroendocrine carcinomas (GI, lung, or pancreatic origin), and advanced, HR+, HER2− breast cancer in combination with exemestane; off-label use in advanced carcinoid tumors, relapsed/refractory Hodgkin lymphoma, advanced/refractory thymoma and thymic carcinoma
- **Dose:** 10 mg once daily with or without food. Dosing with 5 mg if combined with lenvatinib for RCC
- **Half-life:** 30 hours
- **Metabolism:** Major CYP3A4 substrate and P-glycoprotein substrate
- **Side Effects:** Mouth ulcers, rash (acneiform), delayed wound healing, nausea/vomiting, fatigue, anorexia (decreased appetite), cough, shortness of breath, thrombocytopenia, diarrhea or constipation, hypercholesterolemia, HTN, hyperglycemia, anemia, leukopenia
- **Clinical Pearls:** Monitor fasting triglycerides and cholesterol. Levels may increase while on treatment despite the patient's dietary habits. Initiate oral care early on (soft toothbrush, salt, and soda swish).

Futibatinib

- **Alias:** TAS-120
- **Type Mechanism:** An orally bioavailable inhibitor of the FGFR that selectively and irreversibly binds to and inhibits FGFR, which may result in the inhibition of both the FGFR-mediated signal transduction pathway and tumor cell proliferation and increased cell death in FGFR-overexpressing tumor cells. FGFR is an RTK essential to tumor cell proliferation, differentiation, and survival, and its expression is upregulated in many tumor cell types.
- **Drug Class:** FGFR inhibitor
- **Phase:** Phase 3
- **Indications:** Advanced cholangiocarcinoma harboring *FGFR2* gene rearrangements
- **Dose:** 20 mg PO daily
- **Half-life:** ~3 hours
- **Metabolism:** Major CYP3A4 substrate; P-glycoprotein/BCRP substrate
- **Side Effects:** Stomatitis, oral dysesthesia, transaminitis, diarrhea, hyperphosphatemia, constipation, hyperbilirubinemia, hyponatremia, increased lipase, increased CPK, dry mouth, decreased appetite

(Chatila et al., 2020)

Galunisertib

- **Alias:** LY2157299
- **Type Mechanism:** An orally available, small-molecule antagonist of the tyrosine kinase TGF-β receptor type 1 (TGFβR1) that specifically targets and binds to the kinase domain of TGFβR1, thereby preventing the activation of TGF-β–mediated signaling pathways. This may inhibit the proliferation of TGF-β–overexpressing tumor cells.
- **Phase:** Phase 1b/2
- **Indications:** Advanced HCC; unresectable, advanced pancreatic cancer
- **Dose:** 150 mg PO BID for 14 days on, 14 days off for a 28-day cycle
- **Half-life:** 8 hours
- **Side Effects:** Fatigue, thrombosis, dyspnea, thrombocytopenia, lymphopenia, anemia, neutropenia, increased bilirubin, hypoalbuminemia, peripheral edema

(Kelley et al., 2019)

Infigratinib

- **Alias:** BGJ-398
- **Brand:** Truseltiq
- **Type Mechanism:** A selective pan–FGFR kinase inhibitor with activity against

tumors harboring FGFR alterations. It inhibits FGFR signaling and decreases cell proliferation in cancer cell lines with activating FGFR amplifications, mutations, or fusions.

- **Drug Class:** FGFR inhibitor
- **FDA Approval Date:** May 21, 2021
- **Indication:** Unresectable, locally advanced or metastatic cholangiocarcinoma
- **Dose:** 125 mg po daily for 21 days on, 7 days off in a 28-day cycle
- **Metabolism:** Major CYP3A4 substrate, BCRP/ABCG2 substrate, and minor P-gp/ABCB1 substrate
- **Half-life:** 33.5 hours
- **Side Effects:** Hyperphosphatemia, dry eye syndrome, blurred vision, increased lacrimation keratitis, punctate keratitis, and retinal pigment epithelial detachment.
- **Clinical Pearls:** Binds less strongly to FGFR4 so may have less GI toxicity such as diarrhea, liver toxicity, or decrease body weight.

Ipilimumab

- **Alias:** MDX-010; MDX-CTLA4
- **Brand Name:** Yervoy
- **Type Mechanism:** A recombinant human IgG1 mAb that binds to the CTLA4. CTLA4 is a downregulator of T-cell activation pathways. Blocking CTLA4 allows for enhanced T-cell activation and proliferation.
- **Drug Class:** Anti-CTLA4 mAb
- **FDA Approval Date:** March 25, 2011
- **Indications:** Microsatellite instability high (MSI-H) or dMMR mCRC; HCC (in combination with nivolumab); unresectable, malignant pleural mesothelioma; unresectable or metastatic melanoma (in combination with nivolumab); metastatic/recurrent NSCLC with no EGFR or ALK; advanced RCC (in combination with nivolumab)
- **Dose:** Range of dose from 1 mg/kg IV Q 3 weeks, 3 mg/kg IV Q 3 weeks, or 10 mg/kg IV Q 3 weeks, up to 4 doses; NSCLC dose = 1 mg/kg IV Q 6 weeks until PD
- **Half-life:** 15.4 days
- **Side Effects:** Immune-mediated adverse effects (TEN, endocrine disorder, enterocolitis, hepatitis, neuropathy) (black box warning), fatigue, headache, rash/pruritus, nausea/vomiting, diarrhea, abdominal pain, elevated amylase/lipase, elevated ALT/AST, hyperbilirubinemia

Ivosidenib

- **Alias:** AG-120
- **Brand Name:** Tibsovo
- **Type Mechanism:** An inhibitor of IDH1 that inhibits a mutated form of IDH1 in the cytoplasm, which inhibits the formation of the oncometabolite, 2HG. This may lead to both an induction of cellular differentiation and an inhibition of cellular proliferation in IDH1-expressing tumor cells. IDH1, an enzyme in the citric acid cycle, is mutated in a variety of cancers; it initiates and drives cancer growth by both blocking cell differentiation and catalyzing the formation of 2HG.
- **Drug Class:** IDH1 inhibitor
- **FDA Approval Date:** July 20, 2018
- **Indications:** Relapsed/refractory or newly diagnosed AML in adults older than ≥ 75 years with IDH1 mutation
- **Dose:** 500 mg PO daily. Do not take with high-fat meals due to 98% increase in C_{max}.
- **Half-life:** 93 hours
- **Metabolism:** Major CYP3A4 substrate
- **Side Effects:** Fatigue, diarrhea, nausea, decreased appetite, peripheral edema, prolonged QTc, dyspnea, anemia, HTN, transaminitis, leukocytosis due to differentiation syndrome, abdominal pain, skin rash, pruritus
- **Clinical Pearls:** ClarIDHy phase 3 trial demonstrated compelling results for treatment with previously treated, IDH1-mutant cholangiocarcinoma.

Lapatinib Ditosylate

- **Alias:** GSK572016; GW2016; GW-572016
- **Brand Name:** Tykerb
- **Type Mechanism:** Reversibly blocks phosphorylation of the EGFR, HER2, and the ERK1, ERK2, and AKT kinases. Inhibits cyclin D protein levels in human tumor cell lines and xenografts
- **FDA Approval Date:** March 13, 2007
- **Indications:** Metastatic or advanced breast cancer with HER2 overexpression
- **Dose:** 1,250 mg once daily in combination with capecitabine 2,000 mg/m^2 daily, 1,500 mg once daily in combination with letrozole 2.5 mg once daily. Take 1 hour before or 1 hour after meals and avoid grapefruit juice.
- **Half-life:** 24 hours

- **Metabolism:** Major CYP3A4 and P-glycoprotein substrates
- **Side Effects:** Myelosuppression, hand-foot syndrome, liver dysfunction (increased bilirubin, transaminitis), fatigue, nausea/vomiting, diarrhea, rash, decreased LVEF
- **Clinical Pearls:** LVEF should be evaluated in patients before starting therapy, because a decreased EF can occur within the first 9 weeks of treatment. Oral steroids can decrease the levels of the drug and make it less effective. This drug can change the rhythm of the heart. Exercise caution with patients who are already on medications to control irregular heart rhythm.

Larotrectinib

- **Alias:** LOXO-101; TRK inhibitor
- **Brand Name:** Vitrakvi
- **Type Mechanism:** An orally available TRK inhibitor that binds to TRK, thereby preventing neurotrophin–TRK interaction and TRK activation, which results in both the induction of cellular apoptosis and the inhibition of cell growth in tumors that overexpress TRK
- **Phase:** Phase 2
- **Indications:** Relapsed/refractory solid tumors, NHL, or histiocytic disorder with NTRK fusion
- **Dose:** 100 mg PO BID until PD
- **Half-life:** 3.5 hours
- **Side Effects:** Increased transaminases, fatigue, dizziness, anemia, dyspnea, neutropenia, constipation

(Hong et al., 2020; Laetsch et al., 2017)

Lenvatinib Mesylate

- **Alias:** E7080
- **Type Mechanism:** A multitargeted TKI of VEGF receptors VEGFR1 (FLT1), VEGFR2 (KDR), VEGFR3 (FLT4), FGFR1, FGFR2, FGFR3, FGFR4, PDGFRα, KIT, and RET
- **FDA Approval Date:** February 13, 2015
- **Indications:** Differentiated thyroid carcinoma, advanced RCC, or endometrial cancer or unresectable HCC
- **Dose:** 18 mg daily (in combination with everolimus in the RCC); 24 mg daily (thyroid cancer); 20 mg daily in combination with pembrolizumab (endometrial cancer and RCC); 12 mg daily (HCC)
- **Half-life:** 28 hours

- **Metabolism:** Major CYP3A4 substrate
- **Side Effects:** HTN, proteinuria, nausea/vomiting, diarrhea, stomatitis, anorexia, fatigue, QT prolongation, peripheral edema, arthralgia, cough

Lutetium Lu 177 Dotatate

- **Alias:** 177 Lu-DOTATATE; Lutetium Oxodotreotide Lu-177
- **Brand:** Lutathera
- **Type Mechanism:** A beta- and gamma-emitting radionuclide that binds to somatostatin receptors, with highest affinity to subtype 2 receptors (SSRT2); after binding to somatostatin-expressing cells, the lutetium Lu 177 dotatate compound is internalized. Beta-emission induces cellular damage by forming free radicals in somatostatin receptor–positive and surrounding cells.
- **Drug Class:** Radiopharmaceutical
- **FDA Approval Date:** January 26, 2018
- **Indication:** Gastroenteropancreatic neuroendocrine tumors
- **Dose:** 7.4 GBq (200 mCi) every 8 weeks for a total of 4 doses
- **Half-life:** 71 ± 28 hours
- **Side Effects:** Flushing, hypertension, peripheral edema, hyperglycemia, abdominal pain, increased ALT/AST, fatigue, increased SCr, urotoxicity, anemia, lymphocytopenia, neutropenia, thrombocytopenia
- **Clinical Pearls:** Radiation may be detected in the urine for up to 30 days following lutetium Lu 177 dotatate infusion. Caution with family members using same bathroom.

nab-Rapamycin

- **Alias:** ABI-009; nab-sirolimus
- **Type Mechanism:** The macrolide antibiotic rapamycin bound to nanoparticle albumin binds to the immunophilin FKBP-12 to generate a complex that binds to and inhibits the activation of the mTOR, a key regulatory kinase. In turn, inhibition of mTOR may result in the inhibition of the PI3K/Akt pathway and VEGF secretion, which may result in decreased tumor cell proliferation and tumor angiogenesis.
- **Drug Class:** mTOR inhibitor
- **Phase:** Phase 2
- **Indications:** Malignant PEComa, STS (in combination with pazopanib), advanced mCRC (in combination with FOLFOX and bevacizumab)

- **Dose:** 100 mg/m^2 IV Q week for 3 weeks of a 4-week cycle
- **Side Effects:** Mucositis, fatigue, nausea, weight loss, diarrhea, anemia, thrombocytopenia, pneumonitis, transaminitis, hypertriglyceridemia, neutropenia

(Gonzalez-Angulo et al., 2013)

Nivolumab

- **Alias:** BMS-936558; MDX1106; ONO-4538
- **Brand Name:** Opdivo
- **Type Mechanism:** Fully human IgG4 mAb targeting PD-1 receptor on activated T cells
- **FDA Approval Date:** December 22, 2014
- **Indications:** FDA approved for recurrent or metastatic SCCHN, classic Hodgkin lymphoma, unresectable or metastatic melanoma or in adjuvant setting, metastatic NSCLC (nonsquamous), advanced RCC, RCC, HCC, MSI-H CRC, and locally advanced or metastatic urothelial carcinoma
- **Dose:** 3 mg/kg IV Q 2 weeks (H&N cancer, Hodgkin lymphoma, SCLC); 240 mg IV Q 2 weeks or 480 mg IV Q 4 weeks (melanoma, NSCLC, RCC, urothelial cancer, MSI-H CRC, esophageal cancer, HCC); mesothelioma 360 mg IV Q 3 weeks in combination with ipilimumab; combination and then increase it to 3 mg/kg or 240 mg when given alone (HCC, melanoma, RCC)
- **Half-life:** 25 days
- **Side Effects:** Fatigue, nausea, diarrhea, xerostomia, pruritus, immune-mediated colitis, pneumonitis, hyperglycemia, hypertriglyceridemia, hyponatremia, thyroid dysfunction

Octreotide acetate

- **Brand:** Sandostatin
- **Type Mechanism:** Mimics natural somatostatin by inhibiting serotonin release and the secretion of gastrin, VIP, insulin, glucagon, secretin, motilin, and pancreatic polypeptide. It provides more potent inhibition of GH, glucagon, and insulin as compared to endogenous somatostatin. Also suppresses LH response to GnRH, secretion of thyroid-stimulating hormone, and decreases splanchnic blood flow.
- **Drug Class:** Somatostatin analog
- **FDA Approval Date:** October 21, 1988
- **Indication:** Carcinoid syndrome, Gastroenteropancreatic neuroendocrine tumors (VIPomas)
- **Dose:** Initial dosing at 20 mg IM every 4 weeks; may increase to 30 mg IM every 4 weeks or shorter interval of every 3 weeks

- **Metabolism:** LAR is the prefer depot formulation to use in neuroendocrine tumors
- **Half-life:** ~2 hours
- **Side Effects:** Sinus bradycardia, diaphoresis, hyperglycemia, abdominal pain, biliary tract disease, anemia, dizziness, fatigue, arthralgia, flu-like symptoms, and hypothyroidism

Olaparib

- **Alias:** AZD2281; KU-0059436
- **Brand Name:** Lynparza
- **Type Mechanism:** A small-molecule inhibitor of the nuclear enzyme PARP with potential chemosensitizing and radiosensitizing properties
- **FDA Approval Date:** December 19, 2014
- **Indications:** Advanced ovarian cancer, HER2-negative and BRCA mutation breast cancer, MCRPC with HRD, and pancreatic cancer as maintenance therapy after first-line chemotherapy
- **Dose:** 400 mg Q 12 hours. No grapefruit or Seville oranges
- **Half-life:** 11.9 ± 4.8 hours
- **Side Effects:** Nausea/vomiting, leukopenia/lymphopenia, increased creatinine, fatigue, abdominal pain, diarrhea, anemia, thrombocytopenia, muscle pain, infection

Panitumumab

- **Alias:** ABX-EGF; mAb ABX-EGF; rHuMAb-EGFr
- **Brand Name:** Vectibix
- **Type Mechanism:** A fully human mAb that binds specifically to EGFR on both normal and tumor cells and competitively inhibits the binding of ligands for EGFR
- First antibody to demonstrate the use of KRAS as a predictive biomarker
- **FDA Approval Date:** September 27, 2006
- **Indications:** FDA approved for RAS WT mCRC
- **Dose:** 6 mg/kg IV infusion (over 60 or 90 minutes) Q 14 days
- **Half-life:** 7.5 days (range 4–11 days)
- **Side Effects:** Dermatologic toxicity (rash, dermatitis acneiform, pruritus) (U.S. box warning), infusion reactions (fevers, chills, bronchospasms) (U.S. box warning), hypomagnesemia, paronychia, fatigue, nausea/vomiting, diarrhea
- **Clinical Pearls:** Severity of acne-form rash can be minimized with the use of topical

steroid cream, topical antibiotic gel, and doxycycline. Presence and severity of rash may correlate improved response and survival.

(Peeters et al., 2009)

Pazopanib Hydrochloride

- **Alias:** GW786034
- **Brand Name:** Votrient
- **Type Mechanism:** Selectively inhibits VEGFR-1, VEGFR-2, VEGFR-3, FGFR-1, FGFR-3, KIT, and PDGFR, preventing angiogenesis
- **FDA Approval Date:** October 19, 2009
- **Indications:** FDA approved for RCC and STS
- **Dose:** 800 mg daily on fasting stomach, at least 1 hour before or 2 hours after a meal; avoid grapefruit juice
- **Half-life:** 31 hours
- **Metabolism:** Major CYP3A4 substrate
- **Side Effects:** Diarrhea, nausea/vomiting, anorexia, HTN, hair color changes (lightening)
- **Clinical Pearls:** Avoid concurrent medications, which can prolong the QTc interval. Because VEGFR is inhibited, surgical intervention should be avoided.

Pembrolizumab

- **Alias:** MK-3475; SCH 900475
- **Brand Name:** Keytruda
- **Type Mechanism:** A humanized IgG4 mAb directed against human cell-surface receptor PD-1, an inhibitory signaling receptor expressed on the surface of activated T cells. This results in the activation of T-cell–mediated immune responses against tumor cells.
- **FDA Approval Date:** September 4, 2014
- **Indications:** FDA approved for recurrent or metastatic SCCHN, adult and pediatric patients with relapsed or refractory Hodgkin lymphoma, unresectable or metastatic melanoma, adjuvant therapy for melanoma, unresectable or metastatic MSI-H cancers, metastatic NSCLC with PD-L1 expression, or locally advanced or metastatic urothelial carcinoma
- **Dose:** 200 mg IV Q 3 weeks or 400 mg IV Q 6 weeks
- **Side Effects:** Fatigue, rash, hyperglycemia, hypertriglyceridemia, hyponatremia, diarrhea, decreased appetite, anemia, muscle pain, increased SCr, infection, thyroid disorder, immune-mediated pneumonitis

Pemetrexed

- **Alias:** LY231514; MTA
- **Brand Name:** Alimta
- **Type Mechanism:** An inhibitor of TS, DHFR, GARFT, and AICARFT, the enzymes involved in folate metabolism and DNA synthesis, resulting in the inhibition of purine and thymidine nucleotide and protein synthesis
- **FDA Approval Date:** February 4, 2004
- **Indications:** FDA approved for unresectable, malignant mesothelioma in combination with cisplatin and metastatic or locally advanced, nonsquamous NSCLC; off-label use for metastatic bladder cancer, recurrent cervical cancer, platinum-resistant ovarian cancer, and metastatic thymoma
- **Dose:** 500 mg/m^2 IV over 10 minutes Q 21 days. NOTE: Start vitamin supplements with folic acid and vitamin B$_{12}$ 7 days before pemetrexed dose. Give dexamethasone 4 mg PO BID for 3 days, starting 24 hours before pemetrexed dose.
- **Half-life:** 3.5 hours
- **Side Effects:** Fatigue, desquamation, skin rash, nausea, anorexia, vomiting, stomatitis, anemia, neutropenia, edema, transaminitis

Pemigatinib

- **Brand Name:** Pemazyre
- **Type Mechanism:** Oral competitive inhibitor of FGFR1-3 inhibiting FGFR phosphorylation
- **FDA Approval Date:** April 17, 2020
- **Indications:** FDA approved for locally advanced, unresectable, or metastatic cholangiocarcinoma with FGFR2 alteration
- **Dose:** 13.5 mg once daily on days 1 to 14 of a 21-day cycle
- **Half-life:** 15.4 hours
- **Metabolism:** Primarily hepatic through CYP3A4
- **Side Effects:** Edema, hyperphosphatemia, ocular toxicity (retinal pigment epithelial detachment)

(Abou-Alfa et al., 2020)

Pertuzumab

- **Alias:** 2C4; rhuMAb-2C4
- **Type Mechanism:** A humanized recombinant mAb directed against the extracellular dimerization domain of the HER2
- **FDA Approval Date:** June 8, 2012
- **Indications:** FDA approved for HER2-positive breast cancer

- **Dose:** A loading dose of 840 mg IV infusion (over 60 minutes); a maintenance dose of 420 mg IV infusion (over 30–60 minutes) Q 3 weeks; approved to be given in combination with trastuzumab and docetaxel
- **Half-life:** 18 days
- **Side Effects:** Diarrhea, fatigue, neutropenia, rash, nausea/vomiting, stomatitis, embryo–fetal toxicity/cardiotoxicity (U.S. box warning)

Pralsetinib

- **Alias:** BLU-667
- **Brand Name:** Gavreto
- **Type Mechanism:** A next-generation small-molecule RET inhibitor designed to target oncogenic RET fusions and mutations
- **Phase:** Phase 3
- **FDA Approval Date:** September 4, 2020
- **Indications:** Accelerated FDA approval for RET fusion–positive NSCLC and RET fusion or mutation-positive thyroid cancer
- **Dose:** 400 mg PO once daily
- **Half-life:** 16 hours after single dose, 20 hours after multiple doses
- **Metabolism:** Major CYP3A4 substrate

- **Side Effects:** Increased AST/ALT, cytopenias, fatigue, HTN, hypophosphatemia

(Subbiah et al., 2020)

Ramucirumab

- **Alias:** IMC-1121B
- **Brand Name:** Cyramza
- **Type Mechanism:** A recombinant, fully human mAb directed against VEGFR-2. Has a high affinity for VEGFR2, binding to it and blocking the binding of VEGFR ligands VEGF-A, VEGF-C, and VEGF-D to inhibit the activation of VEGFR2, thereby inhibiting ligand-induced proliferation and migration of endothelial cells. VEGFR2 inhibition results in reduced tumor vascularity and growth.
- **FDA Approval Date:** April 21, 2014
- **Indications:** FDA approved for mCRC, advanced or metastatic gastric cancer, metastatic NSCLC, HCC
- **Dose:** 8 mg/kg IV Q 2 weeks (CRC and gastric cancer); 10 mg/kg IV Q 21 days (NSCLC)
- **Half-life:** 14 days
- **Side Effects:** Nausea/vomiting, headache, fatigue, proteinuria, HTN, abdominal pain, DVT

(Tabernero et al., 2015; Wilke et al., 2014)

Regorafenib

- **Alias:** BAY 73-4506
- **Type Mechanism:** Orally bioavailable VEGFR, TIE2, KIT, RAF, RET, PDGFR, FGFR inhibitor
- **FDA Approval Date:** September 27, 2012
- **Indications:** FDA approved for mCRC and unresectable or metastatic GISTs and HCC
- **Dose:** 160 mg PO with food, once daily for the first 21 days of each 28-day cycle
- **Half-life:** 28 hours (range 14–58 hours)
- **Metabolism:** Major CYP3A4 substrate
- **Side Effects:** Hepatotoxicity (U.S. box warning), asthenia/fatigue, diarrhea, anorexia, HTN, mucositis, dysphonia
- **Clinical Pearls:** Assure liver function tests before initiation; monitor blood pressure closely; for diarrhea, prescribe imodium—up to 8 tabs/day. If resistant, first add budesonide 3-mg tab TID, and possibly also add third drug, lomotil, 2 tab four times daily (QID). For mucositis, avoid sodas, acidic fruits, tomatoes, and spicy food. Gargle with baking soda/water mixture am/pm and after each meal. Swish with carafate after baking soda to coat the mouth and protect. May also add viscous lidocaine to assist with diminishing painful eating. For anorexia, add supplemental nutrition to each meal: ensure/boost TID if feasible.

Retifanlimab

- **Alias:** INCMAG012; MGA012
- **Type Mechanism:** A humanized monoclonal antibody directed against the negative immunoregulatory human cell surface receptor PD-1 that binds to and inhibits PD-1 and its downstream signaling pathways. This may restore immune function through the activation of T cells and cell-mediated immune responses against tumor cells.
- **Drug Class:** Anti-PD-1 monoclonal antibody
- **Phase:** Phase 3
- **Indication:** Phase 2 metastatic or unresectable liposarcoma and pancreatic cancer; Phase 2 recurrent gliomas; Phase 2 metastatic urothelial carcinoma; Phase 3 squamous cell anal carcinoma
- **Dose:** Given in combination with chemotherapy with dose of 500 mg IV every 28 days
- **Half-life:** ~11.2 days
- **Side Effects:** Hypothyroidism, skin rash, pruritus, fatigue, diarrhea, asthenia, AST elevation, anemia, palmar-plantar

erythrodysesthesia, pneumonitis, colitis, and abdominal pain
(Rao et al., 2022)

Rucaparib Camsylate

- **Alias:** AG014699; CO-338; PF-01367338
- **Brand Name:** Rubraca
- **Type Mechanism:** The camsylate salt form of rucaparib, an inhibitor of the nuclear enzyme polyadenosine 5′-diphosphoribose PARP, with chemosensitizing, radiosensitizing, and antineoplastic activities. Rucaparib selectively binds to PARP-1, PARP-2, and PARP-3 and inhibits PARP1-mediated repair of single-strand DNA (ssDNA) breaks via the base-excision repair pathway. This enhances the accumulation of DNA strand breaks and promotes genomic instability and apoptosis. Rucaparib may potentiate the cytotoxicity of DNA-damaging agents and reverse tumor cell resistance to chemotherapy and RT.
- **FDA Approval Date:** December 19, 2016
- **Indications:** FDA approved as monotherapy for the treatment of patients with deleterious BRCA mutation (germline or somatic) associated with advanced ovarian cancer in advanced or recurrent setting (as maintenance) and approved for BRCA-mutated MCRPC
- **Dose:** 600 mg BID
- **Half-life:** 17 to 19 hours
- **Side Effects:** Fatigue, increased cholesterol, nausea/vomiting, constipation, decreased appetite, dysgeusia, abdominal pain, thrombocytopenia, anemia, transaminitis, weakness, increased SCr, photosensitivity
(Abida et al., 2020; Jenner et al., 2016)

Sintilimab

- **Brand Name:** Tyvyt
- **Type Mechanism:** Fully human IgG4 mAb that targets checkpoint inhibitor PD-1 and blocks its interaction with PD-L1 and PD-L2; this results in releasing the PD-1 pathway–mediated inhibition of the immune response, including antitumor immune response, thereby decreasing tumor growth
- **Phase:** Phase 3 pending FDA approval
- **Indications:** FDA accepted for review the Biologics License Application (BLA) for sintilimab in combination with pemetrexed and platinum chemotherapy for the first-line treatment of nonsquamous NSCLC chemotherapy
- **Dose:** 200 mg IV Q 3 weeks

- **Half-life:** 35.6 hours
- **Side Effects:** Hypothyroidism, rash, diarrhea, increased liver function tests, pruritis

(Yang et al., 2020)

Sirolimus

- **Alias:** Rapamycin
- **Brand Name:** Rapamune
- **Type Mechanism:** A natural macrocyclic lactone produced by the bacterium *Streptomyces hygroscopicus* that binds to the immunophilin FKBP-12 to generate an immunosuppressive complex that binds to and inhibits the activation of mTOR
- **Indications:** Currently under investigation in phase 1/2 clinical single-agent and combination trials in different cancer types
- **Dose:** 2 mg PO daily maintenance dose following loading; lymphangioleiomyomatosis 2 mg PO daily starting dose (dose titrated per trough concentration)
- **Half-life:** 57 to 63 hours
- **Metabolism:** Major CYP3A4 substrate

- **Side Effects:** Peripheral edema, hypertriglyceridemia, HTN, hypercholesterolemia, creatinine increase, abdominal pain, diarrhea
- **Clinical Pearls:** Monitor fasting triglycerides and cholesterol because levels may increase while on treatment; may consider rapamune-level monitoring.

(Martin Liberal et al., 2012)

Sorafenib

- **Alias:** BAY 43-9006
- **Brand Name:** Nexavar
- **Type Mechanism:** Orally bioavailable inhibitor of RAF, VEGFR, PDGFRβ, and RET
- **FDA Approval Date:** December 20, 2005
- **Indications:** FDA approved for RCC, HCC, and differentiated thyroid carcinoma
- **Dose:** 400 mg PO BID without food (at least 1 hour before or 2 hours after a meal)
- **Half-life:** 25 to 48 hours
- **Metabolism:** UGT1A1 inhibitor; a weak substrate of CYP3A4
- **Side Effects:** Rash, redness, itching, or peeling of skin; alopecia; diarrhea; nausea/vomiting; anorexia; abdominal pain; fatigue

- **Clinical Pearls:** Avoid direct sunlight, use moisturizers after bathing, use mild soap for bathing, and antihistamine for itching. Monitor the patient's blood pressure while on therapy. Instruct the patient on home monitoring. Monitor PTT/INR (International normalized ratio) closely for patients taking Coumadin.

Sotorasib

- **Alias:** AMG510
- **Brand Name:** Lumakras
- **Type Mechanism:** A small molecule that specifically and irreversibly inhibits KRAS G12C through interaction at the P2 pocket, trapping it in the inactive GDP-bound state
- **Phase:** Ongoing phase 3 studies
- **Indications:** Approved in locally advanced or metastatic KRAS G12C-mutated NSCLC
- **Dose:** 960 mg PO once daily
- **Half-life:** 5 hours
- **Metabolism:** CYP3A4 substrate and moderate inducer of CYP3A4
- **Side Effects:** Diarrhea, cytopenias, hepatotoxicity, fatigue, edema, hyponatremia, rash

(Hong et al., 2020; Skoulidis et al., 2021)

Sunitinib

- **Alias:** SU11248
- **Type Mechanism:** Antiangiogenesis inhibitor of PDGFR and VEGFR, as well as KIT and RET
- **FDA Approval Date:** January 26, 2006
- **Indications:** FDA approved in GIST, pNET, and RCC
- **Dose:** 50 mg daily, 4 weeks on treatment followed by 2 weeks off. pNET dose: 37.5 mg daily, continuously without a scheduled off-treatment period
- **Half-life:** 40 to 60 hours
- **Side Effects:** Hepatotoxicity (U.S. box warning), yellowing of skin, fatigue, pyrexia, diarrhea, nausea/vomiting, rash
- **Clinical Pearls:** Swelling of the face, upper, and lower extremities is a possible side effect. Higher risk of complications such as osteonecrosis when taking bisphosphonates with this drug is also possible.

Surufatinib

- **Alias:** Sulfatinib; HMPL-012
- **Type Mechanism:** Small-molecule inhibitor that simultaneously targets tumor angiogenesis (via VEGFR-1, VEGFR-2,

VEGFR-3, and FGFR-1) and immune evasion (via macrophage CSF-1 receptor).

- **Drug Class:** Dual tyrosine kinase inhibitor
- **Phase:** Phase 3
- **Indication:** Phase 3 advanced pancreatic neuroendocrine tumors
- **Dose:** 300 mg po daily for 28 days
- **Half-life:** ~23.3 hours
- **Side Effects:** Hypertension, proteinuria, hypertriglyceridemia, ALT/AST elevations, hyperuricemia, abdominal distention/pain, and diarrhea with rare events: cerebral hemorrhage and GI hemorrhage

(Xu et al., 2020)

Temsirolimus

- **Alias:** CCI-779
- **Brand Name:** Torisel
- **Type Mechanism:** An ester analog of rapamycin that binds to and inhibits mTOR, resulting in a reduced expression of mRNAs necessary for cell-cycle progression and arresting cells in the G1 phase of the cell cycle
- **FDA Approval Date:** May 30, 2007
- **Indications:** RCC
- **Dose:** 25 mg infusion over 30 to 60 minutes once a week. Pretreatment with antihistamine recommended.

- **Half-life:** 17.3 hours
- **Metabolism:** Major CYP3A4 substrate
- **Side Effects:** Rash, asthenia, mucositis, nausea, edema, anorexia, anemia, hyperglycemia, hyperlipidemia
- **Clinical Pearls:** For management of fatigue: Encourage exercise and good sleep hygiene, initiate oral care early on (soft toothbrush, salt, and soda swish), avoid direct sunlight, use moisturizers after bathing, use mild soap for bathing, antihistamines for itching, be aware of possibility of lung toxicity, monitor fasting triglycerides and cholesterol. Levels may increase while on treatment.

Tislelizumab

- **Alias:** BGB-A317
- **Type Mechanism:** A humanized monoclonal antibody directed against PD-1 to prevent PD-1 from binding to the ligands PD-L1 and PD-L2. It is designed to bind less to Fc gamma receptors in order to abrogate antibody-dependent phagocytosis, a mechanism of T-cell clearance and potential resistance to anti-PD-1 therapy.

- **Drug Class:** Anti-PD1 monoclonal antibody
- **Phase:** Phase 3
- **Indication:** Phase 3 NSCLC, hepatocellular carcinoma, and esophageal SCC; Phase 2 urothelial cancer in China
- **Dose:** 200 mg IV every 3 weeks
- **Half-life:** 16.8 ± 5.5 days
- **Side Effects:** Anemia, loss of appetite, nausea, asthenia, pneumonitis, colitis, fatigue, and diarrhea

(Shen et al., 2021)

Trametinib

- **Alias:** GSK1120212; JTP-74057
- **Brand Name:** Mekinist
- **Type Mechanism:** An orally bioavailable molecule that specifically binds to and inhibits MEK1/2
- **FDA Approval Date:** May 29, 2013
- **Indications:**
  - FDA approved for (1) BRAF V600E– or V600K-mutated metastatic melanoma, and (2) in combination with dabrafenib for BRAF V600E–mutated metastatic NSCLC
  - First FDA-approved MEK inhibitor
- **Dose:** 2 mg PO daily
- **Half-life:** 4 to 5 days
- **Metabolism:** Weak CYP2C8 inhibitor and weak/moderate CYP3A4 inducer

- **Side Effects:** Rash or dermatitis acneiform, diarrhea, peripheral edema, fatigue, HTN, transaminitis
- **Clinical Pearls:** To prevent rash, avoid sun exposure and harsh soaps. Encourage patients to avoid spicy and acidic foods. Remain hydrated. Encourage antidiarrheal and antacid medication. Instruct patients to report visual changes immediately. Obtain baseline retinal and retinal vein examination.

Trastuzumab

- **Alias:** Biosimilar ABP 980; biosimilar PF-05280014
- **Brand Name:** Herceptin
- **Type Mechanism:** A recombinant humanized mAb directed against the HER2, inducing an ADCC against tumor cells that overexpress HER2
- **FDA Approval Date:** September 25, 1998
- **Indications:** FDA approved for the treatment of HER2-overexpressing breast cancer in adjuvant or metastatic setting and HER2-overexpressing gastric cancer
- **Dose:** Adjuvant or metastatic breast: Initial dose of 4 mg/kg over 90-minute IV infusion followed by subsequent weekly doses of 2 mg/kg as 30-minute IV infusion. Metastatic gastric: Initial dose of 8 mg/kg

over 90-minute IV infusion followed by 6 mg/kg over 30- to 90-minute IV infusion Q 3 weeks
- **Half-life:** 2 days (for doses <10 mg)
- **Metabolism:** Cardiomyopathy, infusion reactions, embryo–fetal toxicity, and pulmonary toxicity (U.S. box warning); headache; diarrhea; nausea; chills; neutropenia
- **Side Effects:** Infusion reaction common— observe closely during loading dose; LVEF should be evaluated in patients before starting therapy and monitored Q 2 months.

Fam-trastuzumab Deruxtecan

- **Alias:** Anti-HER2 ADC; DS-8201a
- **Brand:** Enhertu
- **Type Mechanism:** A HER2-directed antibody–drug conjugate composed of a humanized IgG1 monoclonal antibody, a cleavable tetrapeptide-based linker, and the cytotoxic component that is a topoisomerase I inhibitor. The deruxtecan component is a cleavable linker and the topoisomerase inhibitor, DXd (an exatecan derivative). Upon binding to HER2 on tumor cells, fam-trastuzumab deruxtecan undergoes internalization and intracellular linker cleavage by lysosomal enzymes, releasing DXd and resulting in DNA damage and cell death.

- **Drug Class:** Anti-HER2 ADC
- **FDA Approval Date:** December 20, 2019
- **Indication:** Unresectable, metastatic breast cancer with HER2-low or HER2 (+); HER2 (+) metastatic colorectal cancer and gastric cancer; HER2 mutant NSCLC
- **Dose:** Breast and NSCLC: 5.4 mg/kg IV every 3 weeks; colorectal and gastric: 6.4 mg/kg IV every 3 weeks
- **Metabolism:** BCRP/ABCG2 substrate; OATP1B1/1B3 substrate; deruxtecan is metabolized through the CYP3A4 pathway
- **Half-life:** 5.4–6.1 days
- **Side Effects:** Neutropenia, decreased LVEF, nausea, vomiting, diarrhea, stomatitis, interstitial lung disease, pneumonitis, alopecia, skin rash, abdominal pain, anemia, ALT/AST elevations, dry eye syndrome, increased serum creatinine, and fatigue
- **Clinical Pearls:** Moderate emetogenic potential

Tremelimumab

- **Alias:** CP-675,206; CP-675; anti-CTLA4 human mAb CP-675,206
- **Type Mechanism:** A human IgG2 mAb directed against the human TCR protein

CTLA4 that binds to CTLA4 on activated T lymphocytes and blocks the binding of the APC ligands B7-1 (CD80) and B7-2 (CD86) to CTLA4, resulting in the inhibition of CTLA4-mediated downregulation of T-cell activation

- **Phase:** Phase 2
- **Indications:** Advanced HCC or biliary tract cancer, TNBC, germ cell tumor, esophageal cancer, urothelial carcinoma (phase 3 global study), high-risk STS, and NSCLC
- **Dose:** 1 mg/kg IV Q 4 weeks for 6 doses, then Q 12 weeks for 3 doses
- **Half-life:** 22 days
- **Side Effects:** Diarrhea, colitis, fatigue, nausea, skin rash, hypophysitis, pruritus

(Comin-Anduix et al., 2016)

Vemurafenib

- **Alias:** RO5185426; PLX4032; RG7204
- **Brand Name:** Zelboraf
- **Type Mechanism:** A PARP-1 and PARP-2 inhibitor with chemosensitizing and antitumor activities. With no antiproliferative effects as a single agent at therapeutic concentrations, ABT-888 inhibits PARPs, thereby inhibiting DNA repair and potentiating the cytotoxicity of DNA-damaging agents.
- **Drug Class:** BRAF kinase inhibitor
- **FDA Approval Date:** August 17, 2011
- **Indications:** Unresectable, metastatic melanoma; Erdheim–Chester disease with BRAF V600 mutation
- **Dose:** 960 mg PO Q 12 hours
- **Half-life:** 57 hours
- **Metabolism:** Major CYP3A4 substrate
- **Side Effects:** Prolonged QT, HTN, peripheral edema, headache, skin rash, neuropathy, fatigue, palmar–plantar erythrodysesthesia, nausea, vomiting, decreased appetite, diarrhea, cutaneous papilloma, SCC of skin, myalgia/arthralgia, increased GGT

Zenocutuzumab

- **Alias:** MCLA-128; Zeno
- **Type Mechanism:** An antibody-dependent cellular cytotoxicity–enhanced anti-HER2xHER3 bispecific antibody. It inhibits HER3 and AKT phosphorylation, induced expression of apoptosis markers, and inhibited growth in chemotherapy-resistant NRG1 fusion–positive metastatic cancer.
- **Drug Class:** Bispecific monoclonal antibody
- **Phase:** Phase 2

- **Indication:** Phase 2 NSCLC, pancreatic cancer, and NRG1 fusion (+) cancers
- **Dose:** 750 mg IV every 2 weeks
- **Half-life:** 4 days
- **Side Effects:** Diarrhea, infusion-related reactions, fatigue, asthenia, anemia
- **Clinical Pearls:** Less GI, skin, and cardiotoxicity

(Schram et al., 2022)

Zolbetuximab

- **Alias:** IMAB362; Claudiximab
- **Type Mechanism:** A chimeric IgG1 monoclonal antibody that specifically binds to CLDN18.2 and mediates cell death through antibody-dependent cellular cytotoxicity and complement-dependent cytotoxicity
- **Drug Class:** Anti-CLDN18.2 monoclonal antibody
- **Phase:** Phase 3
- **Indication:** Phase 3 gastric and gastroesophageal junction adenocarcinoma and pancreatic tumors with moderate to strong CLDN18.2 expression
- **Dose:** Phase 3 dose: 800 mg/m^2 loading dose, followed by 600 mg/m^2 IV every 3 weeks
- **Half-life:** 13–24 days
- **Side Effects:** Nausea, vomiting, fatigue

(Sahin et al., 2021)

Index